THE HUMAN SIDE
OF MEDICINE

THE HUMAN SIDE
OF MEDICINE

Learning What It's Like to Be a Patient and
What It's Like to Be a Physician

Laurence A. Savett, M.D.

Foreword by William H. Harvey

AUBURN HOUSE
Westport, Connecticut • London

Library of Congress Cataloging-in-Publication Data

Savett, Laurence A., 1936–
    The human side of medicine : learning what it's like to be a patient and what it's like to be a physician / Laurence A. Savett.
        p. cm.
    Includes bibliographical references and index.
    ISBN 0–86569–318–8 (alk. paper)—ISBN 0–86569–319–6 (pbk. : alk. paper)
    1. Physician and patient.   2. Medicine—Miscellanea.   3. Medical care—Miscellanea.   I. Title.
    [DNLM: 1. Physician-Patient Relations.   2. Attitude of Health Personnel.
    3. Attitude to Health.   4. Nurse-Patient Relations.   5. Patients—psychology.
    W 62 S266h 2002]
    R727.3.S355   2002
    610.69'6—dc21   2001053837

British Library Cataloguing in Publication Data is available.

Library of Congress Catalog Card Number: 2001053837
ISBN: 0–86569–318–8
          0–86569–319–6 (pbk.)

First published in 2002

Auburn House, 88 Post Road West, Westport, CT 06881
An imprint of Greenwood Publishing Group, Inc.
www.greenwood.com

Printed in the United States of America

The paper used in this book complies with the
Permanent Paper Standard issued by the National
Information Standards Organization (Z39.48–1984).

10 9 8 7 6 5 4 3

Copyright Acknowledgments

The author and publisher gratefully acknowledge permission for use of the photograph and for extensive excerpts from the following material.

Laurence A. Savett, M.D. "Drug-induced Illness: Causes for Delayed Diagnosis and a Strategy for Early Recognition." *Postgraduate Medicine* 67, No. 1 (January 1980): 155–166. Reprinted by permission of *Postgraduate Medicine*.

Laurence A. Savett, M.D. "Medical Care and Teaching: Stories of Inadequacy, Opportunities for Growth." *Primarily Nursing* (January/February 1994): 10–12. Reprinted by permission of *Creative Nursing*.

Laurence A. Savett, M.D., and Susanne G. Savett, M.S.W. "Genuine Collaboration: Our Obligation to Our Patients and to Each Other." *Creative Nursing* (September/October 1994): 11–13. Reprinted by permission of *Creative Nursing*.

Laurence A. Savett, M.D. "Dealing with Uncertainty: Yet Another Dimension in Caring for Our Patients." *Creative Nursing* (January/February 1995): 11–13, 20. Reprinted by permission of *Creative Nursing*.

Laurence A. Savett, M.D. "Spirituality and Practice: Stories, Barriers, and Opportunities." *Creative Nursing*, No. 4 (1997): 7–11, 16. Reprinted by permission of *Creative Nursing*.

Laurence A. Savett, M.D. "How Can I Keep from Becoming Emotionally Involved?" *Creative Nursing*, No. 4 (1998): 3–5. Reprinted by permission of *Creative Nursing*.

Laurence A. Savett, M.D. "Values and Dealing with Change." *Creative Nursing*, No. 3 (2000): 11–13, 15. Reprinted by permission of *Creative Nursing*.

Photograph by Rob Amberg. "Home Health Nurse Examining a Patient in His Home, Madison County, North Carolina." Copyright © 1984. Reprinted with permission of Rob Amberg.

FOR SUE

AND

FOR ALEX AND THE NEXT GENERATION

Teach your children diligently.
Deuteronomy 6:7

I swear . . . that I will fulfill . . . this oath and covenant: . . . to give a share of precepts and oral instruction and all the other learning to my sons and to the sons of him who has instructed me and the pupils who have . . . taken this oath according to the medical law.
The Hippocratic Oath

May I never see in the patient anything but a fellow creature in pain.
Physicians' oath, attributed to Maimonides

Contents

Contents

Tables

Foreword

Dr. Laurence Savett has had a respected career as a practicing physician and medical school teacher. Now retired from active practice, he has dedicated his considerable abilities and energies as an advisor, teacher, and mentor to premedical undergraduates at several institutions. This is an unusual and exciting role for a physician.

Drawing on all these experiences, he has written a most informative book, *The Human Side of Medicine: Learning What It's Like to Be a Patient and What It's Like to Be a Physician*. I enjoyed reading it, and it should be considered required reading for anyone considering a career in medicine. The book is a primer for pre-professional students, including those who are interested but unsure about medicine and those who are firmly committed. It is also a book for medical students and residents, for their teachers and advisors, and for professionals and other staff who work with physicians and patients. It is an important book for patients, who, as Dr. Savett writes in the Introduction, should expect both technical skill *and* humanity from their physicians. I am a strong advocate for responsible *patienthood* and this book reinforces the need for partnering between patient and physician.

Based on many years of practice, Dr. Savett describes what it's like to be a physician, but he details more than the day-to-day tasks performed by the physician. He writes about the dynamics and the potential fragility of the doctor-patient relationship. He addresses issues of compassion, empathy, and sensitivity, using examples collected over his long medical career.

The case studies are wonderful and revealing: the good and bad decisions made, good and bad teaching demonstrated, the rush to judgment underlined, and first impulses discouraged without careful thought. Dr. Savett's life experiences are woven into the fabric of the text, giving the book credibility and warmth.

It is a wonderfully informative book that is all about humanism in medicine. It is well titled, and I like the statement that appears in the book's summarizing chapter: "Good medicine does not just happen; it is thoughtfully planned and practiced." In this context, Dr. Savett's book focuses on thoughtful and careful observations and on reflections free from preconceived biases and prejudices. Emphasis is placed on truly seeing and processing what one is observing, listening, and then, that rare event, hearing what one is listening to. So much of this book is about being a good listener.

This book should be required reading for all medical students, and they should read it more than once, at the beginning of their pre-professional training as undergraduates and frequently during their years in medical school. Today, far too little emphasis is placed on issues of humanity in many medical school curricula. Medical school faculty will be grateful for this text, and they should read it carefully. Advisors who work with undergraduate advisees interested in any area of health care will want to have a copy of this book on their shelves. It is also a useful book around which to build a seminar for pre-professional students, where one might address important questions, such as, "Is a career in medicine a 'humanistic' career supported by science or a 'scientific' career supported by humanism?"

Thank you, Dr. Savett, for focusing on these important issues of humanism in medicine. Your book is greatly appreciated.

William H. Harvey, Ph.D.
Professor of Biology and Chief Health Services Advisor,
Earlham College, Richmond, Indiana
President, Central Association of Advisors for the
Health Professions.

Acknowledgments

"Who are your models? Who are your teachers?"

A career in medicine is a commitment to lifelong learning. I like to ask premeds: "Who are your models? Who are your teachers?" Now I acknowledge my own teachers. Many of them, I am sure, have no idea of the magnitude of their influence.

I learned from many of my patients, who taught me what textbooks do not: nuances of how illnesses behave, how best to say things, the language of compassion, what works and what does not, how people handle tough situations, and about meaning and spirituality. Their stories and their words fill this book. I acknowledge many CanSurmount members who unselfishly shared their stories with my students. I especially thank Carol Lindberg, the coordinator for the St. Paul chapter, who made those connections.

I have felt privileged to teach at the University of Minnesota Medical School since 1969 and at Macalester College since 1994. I continue to learn from my students, and I specifically acknowledge these Macalester students: Alejandro Baigorria, Eric Brown, Robert Carlson, Tierre Christen, Neena Davis, Rebecca Egbert, Cesar Ercole, Paul Evans, Megan Flom, Susannah Ford, Eric Geigle, Marissa Getter, Phung Gip, Laura Goodspeed, Tom Hermanson, Karin Holt, Cara Hummer, Julie Knoll, Nat

Kongtahworn, Anthony Koo, Jessica Maddox, Tarra McNally, Wamaid
Mestey-Borges, Caroline Nerhus, Laura Neumann, Anna Person, Aimee
Powelka, Britta Schoster, Misty Shanahan, Andrea Sternberg, Cathleen
Steinegger, Phang Thao, Jessica Tobin, Kai Tuominen, Amy Voedisch,
and Jeannette Ziegenfuss. Along with many others in the seminar, they
helped me test, refine, clarify, and critique my thought and concepts. I also
acknowledge the insights of two from the University of Minnesota Medical
School: Henry Riter and Ted Haland.

From Bob Feldman, Mike Glasgow, Ruben Haugen, Lou Lachter, Leon
Olenick, Melanie Soucheray, and Chris Volpe—none of them physicians—I gained insight into the question, "What is a professional?"

Later I will allude to my parents' illnesses. Each of them wrestled with serious illness and never gave up. As a participant of their medical dramas, I
learned from them and from my sister Enid what excellent care and
not-so-good care are, and that illness is a family affair. Other family and
friends have told me stories of fine medical care and shameful neglect;
through their eyes, I got more of a picture of what it is like to be a patient or
the family of a patient. Many of their stories appear in the text.

Certain authors influenced my method of practice and teaching. I take
special note of Robert Coles, whom I have never met. His book, *The Call of
Stories*, and his example, that of a physician teaching at an undergraduate
level, gave me the idea for my course at Macalester. And his concept of the
importance of "story," though not new to me, validated and put into the
right words what I had taught for many years.

Years ago I stumbled upon an ad for *Medical Choices, Medical Chances:
How Patients, Families, and Physicians Can Cope with Uncertainty*. The title
tantalized me, and reading the book validated another concept I had continually used but never discussed with others. At my invitation, one of the
authors, Harold Bursztajn, came to St. Paul to discuss his insights in an evening seminar for physicians. From time to time through the years, I have
sent on to him what my students have written about uncertainty and his
text.

My high school history teacher at Utica Free Academy, Frank Mason,
showed me that there is more to learn than what is written. His lectures
presented information and concepts beyond the text, and from him I
learned to examine alternative ways of teaching. For the first time, I realized that there were bad teachers, good ones, and *really* good ones. He was
my first model of a really good teacher. From Otto Liedke, my German professor for four years at Hamilton College, I learned the importance of the
relationship between the student and the teacher and that teaching goes
beyond mastery of a subject; it involves performing. I sometimes find my-

self copying some of his *shtick*, as I hear myself saying to a student, as he would with a smile on his face and a twinkle in his eye, "Mr. X, you being a person of great insight, please tell me. . . ."

The best teacher I have ever had, Earl Schwartz, has taught every member of my family, and I continue to learn from him. He commands an audience with his mastery of the subject, his prose, which is like poetry, the manner of his presentation, and his relationship to his students. He respects his audience, young or old; he never talks down to them. At times he is very, very funny.

Of all the physicians who influenced me, Irving Cramer, my family doctor, had the first and most substantial impact. Whenever I think of the best in a physician, he is my model.

At the University of Rochester School of Medicine and Dentistry, George Engel helped to fashion my approach to patients. He took the hard-to-define qualities of the human side of medicine, described them in detail, refined them as they applied to each patient, taught that the psychosocial history ought to be part of every transaction, placed those skills as a central part of the curriculum, and then modeled it for us by teaching us clinical interviewing. Our first experience with patients, whether it was on a medical or surgical ward, was overseen by him and his colleagues in the medicine-psychiatry liaison section of the faculty.

Two of my teachers at Cleveland Metropolitan General Hospital were especially influential. Lawrence Weed devised "the problem-oriented medical record," actually a system of reasoning, which helped me organize my diagnostic and therapeutic impressions on paper. That discipline focused my inquiry and pursuit of clues from the patient's story and streamlined my thinking. I used it throughout my career in practice, and it is a wonderful teaching tool. V. N. Kapur, a pulmonary specialist, taught me how to read chest x-rays. Long before the advent of CT scans, he saw clues in plain x-rays that no one else saw, and he taught me how to discover those clues. In providing me a system of approaching an abnormal x-ray in a stepwise fashion, he also taught me to transfer that approach to other clinical situations.

My senior associate in Gloucester, Walter O'Donnell, a fine primary care internist, writer, and student of the sociology of medicine, taught me the best way to say difficult things to patients. He relished telling me his patients' stories as he signed out to me on a weekend, and he enjoyed hearing about mine. The maxim "90 percent of patients' problems are within the ken of 90 percent of most doctors" came from him. He also showed me how to run an office efficiently. He dictated all his notes, had his secretary transcribe them sequentially and in duplicate, placed them in the patient's chart, and kept the copy, essentially a diary of his professional day, as a resource in his writing. Throughout my practice, I followed that example; and a diary of one of my days provides the content of chapters 8 and 22.

It was my special privilege in Gloucester to learn from Warren Babson, the dean of Gloucester medicine, a meticulous surgeon, consummate diagnostician, and perpetual teacher. I remember vividly the moment when he consulted on my patient with a perforated duodenal ulcer, beckoned me to the bedside, and said, "Listen to this, a hepatic friction rub," a rare physical finding, diagnostic of the intraabdominal perforation I had suspected. He taught me about collaboration, about defining the roles of each physician in the care of their common patient, that sometimes taking a chance in treatment, despite uncertainty, is necessary. I liked to watch him deal softly, firmly, and credibly with patients, colleagues, and hospital staff. His credentials were his experience and his commitment to his patients, to the Addison Gilbert Hospital, and to the community at large.

Gordon Addington, another surgeon, also an ordained minister and former missionary, was my St. Paul physician-soulmate. We shared the care of many patients and also shared our views about meaning in medicine and other spiritual matters. I continue to accumulate role models. Denis Clohisy, a University of Minnesota orthopedist, sustained my wife and me with his humanity as we dealt with the pain and the uncertainty of a complex illness in 1997.

My friend Vicki Itzkowitz, a writer and editor, helped me define the audience for this book and its content and purpose. She helped me see that even if the book were never published, nonetheless the writing of the book—the drafting, revising, recomposing—would be a labor of love and self-discovery. If lifelong learning is an important quality of a career in medicine and, as a medical school applicant taught me, one dimension of lifelong learning is "learning more about yourself," then the writing of this book has been an end in itself.

When I was exploring new ways to stimulate myself professionally, my friend Marie Manthey, a very creative thinker, nurse, administrator, teacher, and consultant, well known for her concept of "primary nursing," suggested I write the first of several articles for the journal Creative Nursing. By recruiting me for its editorial board, she enhanced my appreciation of the partnership between physicians and nurses.

Many reviewed all or parts of this manuscript. They rewarded me with their candor, an important part of any relationship. I thank Ruth Cope, Earl Schwartz, Paul Evans, Lou Lachter, Marie Manthey, Walter O'Donnell, Vicki Itzkowitz, Jonathan Spira-Savett, Bob Feldman, Martha Palmer, Chris Bliersbach, and Annie Birnbaum. I thank Gregory

Vercellotti, Madgetta Dungy, and Ilene Harris from the University of Minnesota Medical School; Susan Resnik at the University of California, San Diego, School of Medicine; my colleague pre–health profession advisors at Macelester and the University of St. Thomas, Lin Aanonsen, Jan Serie, Rebecca Hoye, Darlane Kroening, and Charlotte Ovechka; and my fellow advisors at other institutions, Heidi Lang, William Harvey, Karen Paulsen, and Barbara Huntington.

Lisa Legge and I had collaborated on material for *Creative Nursing*, and she consented to review this manuscript critically. She unraveled and reshaped complicated sentences, helped me sharpen the text and clarify my thoughts, and did so with good humor and respect—other qualities of a good relationship. She would be a fine doctor and teacher. I learned a lot from her.

David Unowsky helped me focus on the logistics of getting the book into print. Through Susan Resnik and Elizabeth Kramer, I met John Harney, who gave me realistic advice about content, length, and marketing and made the connection with Greenwood Publishing Group. Jane Lerner, my production editor at Greenwood, coordinated the task of turning my manuscript into a finished work and patiently shepherded me through the process, no small job.

For the use of his photograph, "Home health nurse examining a patient in his home, Madison County, North Carolina," I thank my friend and teacher, Rob Amberg. Rob lives in Madison County and has documented its rural life over the years with his poignant photographs and sensitive text.

Through the years, my daughter, Ellen, has kept me humble. Never reluctant to critique my teaching style, question my views, or shore me up with the wisdom of a younger person, she helped me examine some long-held opinions. A skilled librarian, she has pointed me to good resources and encouraged me to hone my own research skills. Since he was very young, my son, Jon, has stimulated me with his insights, his sense of humor, and his intellectual prodding. As a rabbi and high school teacher, he has provided yet another model of good pedagogy and has helped me to examine the similarities between the doctor-patient relationship and the teacher-student one. Both kids are very good writers. Both take me seriously, but not too seriously.

Finally, there is Sue. Through the years, my wife has helped me refine how I speak with patients and colleagues and struggle with how to establish rapport with patients with whom I am having difficulty. When I have struggled in other ways—with a patient in failing health, with relationships, or with life's more serious dilemmas—she has helped me sort things out.

Much of the wisdom related to dealing with patients comes from the social work paradigm, which she helped me understand. Her profession and mine overlap nicely, and together we now teach first-year medical students. Sue taught me most about relationships; ours continues to grow. Many, many times, I tell others, "Sue is the best part of me."

Introduction: Defining the Human Side of Medicine and Identifying the Audience

"The patient is the center of the drama."

At a time of great changes in the technology and delivery of medical care, what is timeless and unchanging for patients and physicians is the human side of medicine, the nontechnical part. Many feel that unless one is by nature a compassionate and understanding person, that dimension of medicine is hard to teach and hard to learn.

Two premises inspired this book and the course of the same name that I teach at Macalester College, a small nationally known liberal arts college in St. Paul, Minnesota, that it is as important for a physician to master the human side of medicine as its technology and that the human side of medicine can be taught. Attending to the human side enhances care. Again and again, elements of the human side hold the key to diagnosis and treatment by recognizing the unique qualities of each patient. Attending to the human side of medicine enriches the experience for all those in the caring professions.

Some years ago, I was a guest in a class of adult students of a world-renowned biblical scholar. When they asked him to eulogize a recently deceased colleague, equally well known, they expected high praise. Instead he was critical. "He didn't leave even one person to carry on his work," he said. "He created a private language that was not transferable. It was opaque and so it was not useful to others. Transparent knowledge can be used by others and can be transmitted. There are those who do what they do well, but it is not teachable. He gave solutions but not formulas, and formulas can be used by others."

In this book, I reflect on "formulas" for the human side of medicine, based on over thirty years of practice and of teaching, mentoring, and advising medical students and undergraduates. I describe them so that others can use them as students, practitioners, teachers, and informed patients. I suggest "transparent" formulas for thoughtful medical interviewing, exploring the psychosocial issues related to illness, addressing uncertainty, collaborating, developing relationships, attending to values, and for integrating all of these skills into preparation for a career's worth of good patient care.

The Human Side of Medicine describes what keeps the practice of medicine stimulating: not fascinating cases, but fascinating people—the best reason to enter medicine. Attention to the human side is the physician's best protection against professional disenchantment. The book validates the relationship between physician and patient as crucial to all that transpires between them; it is not simply a vestige of "the good old days." It integrates science and technology with the human side but declares that knowledge of science is not enough if one is to be a good physician. The human side of medicine is not simply "being nice to patients"; it is a combination of many dimensions of care, a deliberate, focused, reproducible process. Its elements can be analyzed, and most anything that can be analyzed can be taught. I continued to analyze and learn as I wrote this book.

I know that the human side of medicine can be taught, because I learned about it from other physicians, nurses, psychologists, social workers, clergy—and from patients, an almost infinite number and the real experts. As physicians, we have an obligation to the community of patients, to colleagues, to prospective physicians, and to teachers to share and teach what we do in a way that is attractive, interesting, transmittable—and transparent. Then the teacher-student relationship becomes a model for the doctor-patient relationship.

THE AUDIENCE

The Human Side of Medicine addresses a primary audience of students already committed to a career in medicine, those just beginning to consider it, those who counsel them, and physicians-in-training in medical school and residency training programs. It also speaks to experienced physicians, nurses, social workers, clergy, and others in the clinical professions, to those who teach medicine, to those who work with doctors and patients in hospitals and physicians' offices, and to patients.

The Human Side of Medicine *addresses students already committed to a career in medicine and those beginning to consider it and wondering what it is like.* It is a recruiting book, intended to attract talented, compassionate people to the profession. Though this is not a book about tactics in applying to medical school, it will enhance the reader's understanding of a medical career and help the process of applying by focusing the student on the essential elements of being a physician. Among the most important choices in life is that of a career and life's work. In this single choice are combined our values and aspirations, our self-expectations and assessment of our talents, uncertainty, consideration of costs—time and money, and concern about how the choice will have impact on our personal and family life. The choice is, in a word, complex. The choice of a medical career is all of that.

This book is intended to provide fundamental information and perspective about the experience of being a patient and a physician in a way that is rarely taught at the undergraduate level, so that students can make an informed choice, the first step toward a satisfying career. The book will help those who have thought about a medical career for the right reasons—the desire to serve and the intellectual challenge—but declined serious consideration for invalid ones. One is that the current system of medical care, especially managed care, intrudes inappropriately on the relationship between patient and physician and the amount of time spent together. Regardless of their practice setting, physicians who have always put their patients' interest first and never compromised their professional values have preserved their identity and enthusiasm as caring doctors. Attending to the human side of medicine does not take much time, and it is time well spent. The book should help to dispel other myths: that physicians can not have a personal life and that it takes a genius to be a doctor.

This book is for those who are already learning how to be physicians in medical schools and residency training programs. For those in the first years of medical school, it will provide an ongoing context for learning about the human side of medicine. For those in the clinical years and the residency beyond, it will enlarge and reinforce what they have learned. I have set out to write for them a book full of stories to create a warm anticipation of the joy of a medical career.

This book is for physicians, those in practice or retirement and those who may be struggling with change or disenchantment. It is directed also to those who never had the opportunity to talk—*really* talk—with a colleague about what it is like to be a physician and the meaning of the career. By validating the physician's commitment to the human side of medicine, I hope to reinforce the joy of recognition and to rekindle that joy for those who, in the midst of day-to-day pressures, may have forgotten the real reason why they chose that career—for the human side. In the course of this writing, I have, of course, heightened my own joy. The book is meant to model the role of reflection on one's career; such an activity can be satisfying and renewing, like a "sabbatical in place." The book is also meant to encourage physicians to recycle their experience by teaching and modeling it for students.

This book is for teachers of medicine, those who are good at it, those who wish they could do it better, and those who would like to examine what works in teaching and what does not. Not many of us who teach medicine have had formal training as educators or speak regularly with our fellow teachers about effective techniques. As teachers describe, understand, and reflect on what they do in caring for patients and teaching others, they can better critique, sharpen, discard, reproduce, and improve their techniques and teach them. Medical school curricula are often long on teaching disease states and short on teaching the human side of medicine.

This book is for other professionals—nurses, physical and occupational therapists, psychologists, social workers, chaplains and other clergy—and staff who work with patients and their families in hospitals, physicians' offices, nursing homes, and patients' homes. By enhancing their appreciation of what it is like to be a patient and a physician, they will see even more clearly the opportunities to work together and serve patients better.

Finally, *this book is for patients.* This book will help them recognize good care and affirm that they need not choose their physicians either for their humanity or for their technical skill; they can expect both. Older patients remember what it was like to have a physician who knew them well, over a long period of time, who appreciated their place in their family and in their community, who asked what was going on in their lives, and who could integrate that knowledge into the decisions made and advice offered. Other patients may not know that they can expect both technical excellence and humanity. By understanding how their physicians work, patients can be more effective partners in their own care.

This book, in short, is for all of us kindred souls. The goals are common to us all.

THE PHYSICIAN EXPERIENCE: AN INTRODUCTION

Physicians have the privilege to serve in ways that few careers allow. Patients and their families depend on us, by sharing their burdens and often by turning their burdens over to us completely.

Being a physician is a joy. The intellectual stimulation of dealing with people and their problems, simple and complex, and the variety of challenges is exhilarating. Sobering, too, for patients share the stories of their lives, given only the simplest of encouragement: "How is this for you?" or "What's going on in your life?" Such questions give them permission to tell their stories.

Each patient has a story, and few are reluctant to tell it. When I ask, "Who do you share your feelings with?" many will answer, "My wife (or husband or uncle or friend)," but more than you can imagine will say, "You're the only person I've ever told about this."

So being a physician—privilege and joy aside—is a responsibility. If we are to be partly responsible for the physical and psychological problems of our patients, we must know what we are doing. We must know what to look for, how to get the information, how to identify all the issues, how to discard the trivial, how to use the technology of medicine (and how to restrain ourselves from using it unnecessarily), how to address issues of ethics and uncertainty, and how to integrate all of this information and knowledge quickly into action that serves our patients well.

Physicians are perpetual teachers. We teach our patients; uninformed, they are less likely to follow our instructions. We teach our colleagues also; each consultation, formal or informal, is an opportunity to teach. Many of us teach in medical schools, residency programs, and a few, like me, in undergraduate settings. We are also perpetual students. We learn from our teachers and our colleagues, from what we read and hear in the medical milieu, from our patients, and from our students. We learn from our experience within and outside of our careers. A career in medicine is a commitment to lifelong learning.

But because medicine is changing, the community faces the hazard that attention to the human side of medicine may be neglected. Of all the letters of appreciation I received from patients during my years of practice, not one thanked me for "that great CT scan," "that great blood test," or "that great surgical referral." Rather, they expressed gratitude for my listening, being present, helping them through difficult times, providing emotional support, and enabling them to understand what was going on and how to deal with it—all aspects of the human side of medicine. Patients ought to expect that from all their physicians.

Many argue that unless one is by nature a compassionate and understanding person, the human side of medicine is hard to teach. Not so. I believe that exposing undergraduates to that aspect of a medical career should help attract talented and compassionate people to the profession and provide a context for lifelong learning. I also believe that teaching the human side of medicine as a primary, and not incidental, subject in medical school and that continuing to emphasize it throughout postgraduate residency training is critical to becoming a good doctor. The community of patients is the ultimate beneficiary. Absent the human side, both patients and their physicians lose.

I am a primary care physician, an internist trained before the advent of the major technologic advances in medicine. I learned medicine at the University of Rochester in upstate New York, a medical school whose curriculum was firmly based in the biopsychosocial view of illness. I have had good physicians as models. I have been a patient, a concerned family member, and I am the husband of a talented and compassionate medical social worker. All of these influences contribute to how I look at the doctor-patient relationship.

I am also a perpetual student. I am accustomed to asking, "What did I learn from this encounter with the patient? What did I learn from this class that I taught? From this student?" The insights from these sources make me a better physician and teacher.

My ongoing experience as a teacher is threefold. I have taught medical students, interns, and residents for thirty years at the University of Minnesota, and during most of those years, I have taught small groups of first- and second-year medical students in one of their first direct experiences with patients, as they are beginning to form their habits of practice. Though the course was designed to teach them skills in medical interviewing and diagnosis, I added dimensions emphasizing the human side of medicine. In the last eight years, I have taught undergraduates at Macalester College. The course is called, "Seminar in the Human Side of Medicine: What It's Like to Be a Patient; What It's Like to Be a Physician." And finally, each day of my practice, I taught my patients the meaning and implications of their illness and treatment. One of our roles as physicians is to transmit the best of what we have learned, to build on those lessons, and to preserve the timeless values. A statement in rabbinic literature declares, "We may not be able to finish the task; even so, we shouldn't shrink from it."[1]

My generation of physicians—I am in my 60s and graduated medical school in 1961—is especially important as a bridge generation. Our teachers were educated before the arrival of big medical technology—fiberoptic endoscopy, coronary artery catheterization, CT and MRI scanners, even blood chemistry screening tests—and so they relied a great deal on the medical interview, the patient's story of illness. They valued it as the entrée to the patient's diagnosis and treatment and squeezed more information out of it. They thought things over as much as possible before pressing on to laboratory work or consultations. They recognized the value of presence.

Less reliant on technology, they were better listeners. Treatment in those days was simpler also. The therapeutic choices often included no treatment, simple treatment such as penicillin for infection or digitalis for congestive heart failure, time, or rest. There were no intensive care units or "extraordinary measures" like ventilators, cardiopulmonary resuscitation, and dialysis.

Wherever I practiced, there were always one or two extraordinary physicians, people with unique viewpoints and approaches and extra measures of diagnostic and therapeutic wisdom. Colleagues recognized them as community treasures and resources. When, despite their own best efforts and those of their consultants, physicians still did not know what was going on with a patient and what to do next, they turned to one of them. Most of the time, they came up with the solution to the unsolved diagnostic problem not by collecting more laboratory data, but simply by reinterviewing the patient, reviewing the other material, and looking at all the information in a different way. When they taught their "method," they did it by "thinking out loud," by making their process "transparent."

Similarly, I have had other remarkable teachers, inside and outside of medicine, noteworthy not only for *what* they taught me but also for *how* they taught and how they organized and presented their material. When these people, master clinicians and teachers, retired or died, they took many of their secrets with them, a loss to the community of patients and physicians. Would it not have been great for them to have been debriefed and to have had their skills and secrets described, sorted out, and published?

To a certain extent, this book is my attempt to debrief myself. Not that I am extraordinary in the way that I have described these others. Nonetheless, I reflect on these matters, and, through the years, I have kept good records, not only of clinical data, but also of how patients, students, and teachers say things. I have recorded how I say things to patients and students and what works and does not work.

Lest we forsake the best of the past as we move to the future, we should recognize that medicine, like the Talmud, a compendium of biblical commentary and discussion, "is built layer upon layer, the result of the combined labors of many generations. . . . The creative work of one generation serves as the basis for the creative work of the next.[2] . . . [It] is thus the recorded dialogue of generations of scholars [and] has all the characteristics of a living dialogue."[3] If we do not continually write about, clarify, integrate, and carry on the "dialogue" of medicine, then we do not build on prior knowledge, and we are condemned forever to reinvent the wheel. Our task, as physicians and teachers who appreciate the importance of the human side of medicine, is to preserve those values and techniques and pass them on to our students.

TEACHING THE HUMAN SIDE OF MEDICINE

Many patients, students, and friends have expressed doubt that the human side of medicine can be taught. "Either you have it or you don't," they say. Unequivocally I declare: "The human dimensions of medicine and how to apply that knowledge can be taught—by drawing upon students' own experiences, by modeling the relationship, and by thoughtful examination of the infinite number of medical transactions."

My undergraduate, semester-long course at Macalester College, "Seminar in the Human Side of Medicine: What It's Like to Be a Patient; What It's Like to Be a Physician," meets in a two-hour weekly session, with discussions, weekly papers, and a term paper. Together the students and I explore the essence of that part of medicine, seen from the standpoint of the patient and the physician. Let me parse the title of the course.

The course is a *seminar*, not a lecture course. That means that there is an intimacy between my students and me, which allows for open and open-ended discussion. Nonetheless, there are a framework and an agenda to the discussions, which this book approximates. During the seminar meetings, we often tell stories from our own lives and use these stories as data for our discussion.

The human side of medicine: The theme of the course, and of this book, is that medicine, while technical in many of its methods, is a human profession, about people. While illness may be defined in terms of an abnormal organ or organ system, it is ultimately about human distress, and the science of it is only part of the method of inquiry and action. It does not always help the patient when the physician presents technical information without providing context, comfort, compassion, and continuity—all human dimensions of medicine.

What it's like to be a patient takes priority in the subtitle over what it's like to be a physician. The primary axiom of the course and of my practice and professional life is "the patient is the center of the drama," not the doctor, not the hospital, not the insurance company or other institution. The task of the physician is to appreciate *what it's like* to be in the patient's situation, to clearly define the patient's needs, and then to help the patient meet those needs. That is where we begin the course.

The composite life of a physician, *what it's like to be a physician*, cannot be ignored by anyone considering a career in medicine. Being a physician means dealing not simply with illness but with people with illness, having to interpret and decode their stories in order to define their problems before one can suggest and provide a remedy. That is a very stimulating and satisfying activity. *What it's like to be a physician* is more than *what the doctor does all day*. It means knowing how to plan our day to make best use of time, to integrate our professional and personal lives and provide balance, to set limits, to attend to our family, and to share some of the emotional burdens. Being a physician is intense work, filled with complex decisions (most of which become second nature with experience), and we can be easily seduced into allowing our professional activity to overtake our personal life.

We begin the course with a story of one patient's experience with illness. To this we add stories from the students' experiences, for almost all students have had experience with either their own or a close family member's encounter with a more than trivial illness. We learn from stories. Sometimes we miss all their lessons. Sometimes we unconsciously alter them by how we listen or how we retell them. But this does not negate the point that one of the joys and opportunities of being a physician is being privy to stories and the discovery that is involved.

I like to use the photograph on page xxxiv when I teach the course. "Take three minutes to study the photo," I tell the students, "and then take ten minutes to write a story about it." All they know for sure is the caption: "Home health nurse examining a patient in his home, Madison County, NC." Each of the students' stories, of course, is different, focusing variously on the man, the woman, the nurse, or all three. The students construct stories of differing acute and chronic illnesses; the man's various losses—health, independence, income, and ultimately life; and the impact of his illness on the man, the woman in the doorway, usually called "his wife," and the nurse. Some notice the photo of the serviceman on the bookshelf in the background, and construct yet another story. Some notice the walker in the foreground. Others notice the modesty of the dwelling.

After the students read their stories to the whole class, I tell them what the phogorapher, Rob Amberg, told me. "The woman to the right is the man's daughter. He was 94 years old when the photograph was made, and he had been living with her and her husband for a number of years. The home health nurse made regular weekly visits with him. That work is incredibly rewarding. The nurses play a vital role in our very rural, often isolated community, acting not only as interpreters between patients and clinic doctors, but also as a strong social connection. Most of the nurses end up being good friends with their patients. Both the man and his daughter are long gone, and, while I'm sure he would be flattered to be thought so young, I suspect she would be equally upset to be thought so old,"

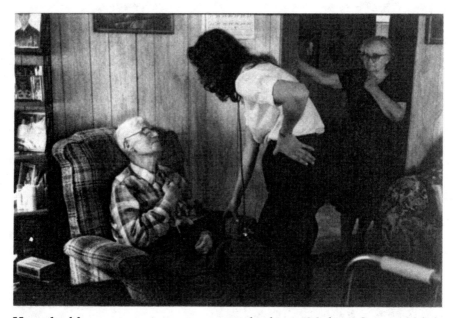

Home health nurse examining a patient in his home, Madison County, North Carolina. Shot for *Southern Exposure* magazine. Photographer: Rob Amberg. Copyright © 1984.

The photograph is but a moment in these people's lives. The point of the exercise is to demonstrate that we unconsciously construct stories about people from scant knowledge of the facts and then draw conclusions from those stories. The less we know for sure, the more inaccurate our inferences. Especially as physicians and other health care professionals, we need to know as much of the story as possible to make valid decisions and do our jobs well.

I have set out to write a sweet book, full of patients,' students', and physicians' stories and reflections. It represents the cumulative wisdom of all my teachers—my professors, my colleagues, my family and friends, and my patients and students. Much of what I do and much of who I am as a physician and teacher is derived from what I have learned from them.

I'll begin chapter 1, after presenting the medical *history*, by telling a *story*. Then I will identify the *issues*, address the role of the *doctor-patient relationship*, and finally ask, "*What did I learn?*"

PART I

WHAT IT'S LIKE TO BE A PATIENT

Chapter 1

Medical Care Starts with the Patient's Story

"The story is never over."

One cannot be a good physician without understanding what it is like to be a patient.

THE HISTORY

A 50-year-old physician had chest pains for two months, brought on by exertion and relieved by rest. His physical examination was normal. A cardiac stress test was positive: Walking on the treadmill reproduced his pain, and the change in the electro-cardiogram pattern indicated that the pain was from coronary insufficiency, impaired circulation of blood to the heart. A coronary angiogram, an x-ray of the arteries of the heart, showed multiple areas of coronary artery narrowing. A few days later, he had coronary artery bypass surgery. Three days following surgery, he had a three-hour period of extremely rapid heartbeat, a disturbance of cardiac rhythm called "atrial fibrillation with rapid ventricular response," associated with chest pain and hypotension, a drop in blood pressure; it resolved with treatment. He was discharged from the hospital eleven days after the surgery, recovered uneventfully, and returned to work part-time in ten weeks and full-time six weeks after that.

This medical history, equivalent to a brief oral case presentation or to a note in a patient's chart, summarizes the story of a real illness.

Is it the whole story? And if not, is it sufficient to describe what the patient and his family went through? And if there is a longer story, is appreciation of that saga important in knowing how to care for the patient and his family?

What can we learn from knowing the whole story?

THE STORY

The patient kept a journal of his memories of this period in his life. Here is the story in his own words.

I had had pain in my lower teeth on vigorous exertion for many years. I recall that even playing touch football twenty years ago had brought it on. So when I noticed it again, I didn't pay much attention to it. "It's simply more of the same," I thought, "unlikely to be of consequence."

For two months though, beginning in May, I noticed that besides the pain in my teeth, I would have pain, not severe, high up in my chest and in my left arm with certain activities such as walking in the park with my son and walking across the street from my office to the hospital. The pain would promptly go away, so how serious could it be, I thought. To validate that point, I would climb three or four flights of stairs. Always the last flight would bring on the pain. I would fall asleep at night thinking about it, wake up in the morning thinking about it, and always say to myself, "It's not my heart." I told no one, not even my wife, in whom I confide everything.

And then in July, after two months of this, I said to myself, "It's not just me who depends on me, but also my wife and my two children," and "My children are both going away in the next two months, one to study abroad for a year and the other to Boston, 1,400 miles away, to start college. If I am really ill, it would be unfair to spring this on them from a distance." And finally, I asked myself, "What would I advise *me* if I saw *myself* as a patient?"

So I made an appointment for a stress test to be done two days later. Then I told my wife about the pains and the test. And, doing my best to deny that this could be anything serious, on the night before the stress test, I called a friend in Boston to tidy up plans for a vacation later that month. I saw my personal physician the morning of the test and told him about my symptoms for the first time. I kept believing that I would pass the test.

The doctor who monitored the test stopped it after two minutes. I knew that meant that the test was positive, and she confirmed my fear. I returned to my personal physician who by then had been informed of the results. He prescribed nitroglycerin to be used in an emergency and arranged for me to see a cardiologist two days later.

My wife picked me up at the office. I told her the results. My voice broke and I wept. Later I spoke to my children, telling them for the first time what was going on.

That evening I told my office partner. The next day I worked and saw patients. "Why not?" I reasoned. "It will be an easy day—no especially difficult problems." But I was preoccupied and couldn't concentrate. At the end of the day, I told my staff, and again my voice broke. But even then I was tentative about how long I'd be away—the stress test might be falsely positive.

The next day, Friday, I did not work. With my wife I saw the cardiologist. The coronary angiogram had already been arranged for the following Monday, and I asked that I be the first case of the day, in order to avoid delays or postponement, common occurrences on a busy cardiology service.

Whom else did I tell? My rabbi, with whom I had a close relationship and friendship. My father, 81, healthy but emotionally vulnerable and living in another city. My sister, a nurse, also living elsewhere.

My father's immediate response was, "I'll be there tomorrow." I was annoyed that he decided without asking me and I asked him not to come until we knew the results of the angiogram. Later he called back and said, "Tell me what you want me to do."

What did I feel? Sadness. "I'd hate to lose me," I thought. "I'm a helluva guy." And shame, that I didn't take good enough care of myself, that I wasn't "a jock."

The following day, Saturday, I went to our synagogue, a small congregation. In my behalf, the rabbi said the special prayer one says for an ill person, asking for "healing of body and healing of spirit." I had mixed feelings about acknowledging to those gathered that I was not well. On the one hand, I wanted the support of my congregation; on the other hand, I was embarrassed by my illness.

The next day, I attended a previously scheduled gathering of my wife's family. By then my problem was no secret, and they all gave me their moral support. One had had a similar problem with a good outcome. His suggestion: "Get another opinion."

On Monday, I entered the hospital for the angiogram. A lot was running through my mind. Should I take the pills routinely prescribed before an angiogram? What's the test *really* like? Could it harm me? What's the outcome going to be? The test went easily enough.

That day, the cardiologist came to my room to discuss the findings. He told my wife and me that there were a number of narrowed arteries and their branches, that the situation was serious, and that he was uncertain if surgery would help. We were stunned!

My children, who had been part of this drama since the previous week, had been sent out of my room by the cardiologist for what we thought would be a brief talk with us. That talk lasted over half an hour. When they returned, they were outraged at having been excluded. "Don't ever do that again!" they said.

The next day the surgeon arrived and said that surgery *was* an option and that he could do it. With the cardiologist, I examined my choices. Treatment with medicine alone would not improve the long-term outlook. Angioplasty, using a balloon-tipped catheter to enlarge the areas of narrowing, might be a possible remedy but had its risks. Surgery, though also risky, seemed the best choice.

We agreed to proceed with the surgery. Of each of my physicians, the internist, the cardiologist, and the surgeon, I asked for continuity of care, that each would see me daily and be personally available, rather than a surrogate. I did not want decisions about my care to be made by someone who did not have a complete perspective about me medically. I wanted to be looked after by someone who knew who I was. I did not want too many cooks spoiling the broth. I did not want to feel abandoned. They agreed.

Then I went home to await surgery, scheduled for the following Friday. Again I requested that I be the first case of the day.

In the interim I arranged my affairs. Though I felt things would turn out well, I approached the event by planning for the possibility that I might not survive. With my wife and my attorney, a close friend, I reviewed my will, my assets, my personal and office financial matters, and my insurance, and I made sure that my wife had access to all of this material. I was struck by my wife's strength. I wrote individual letters to my wife, to my son and daughter, and to my father and sister. Before the surgery, I gave each the letter. These were not letters "to be opened in the event of my death" but rather ones to be read immediately (and maybe more than once), expressions of love, affection, and admiration, validating our relationships. I occupied myself with many tasks. I "faced my mortality."

On Thursday, early in the day before surgery, I checked into the hospital. In the course of interviewing me, the admissions clerk inquired about how much cash I was carrying: "Do you have any money?" Never one to pass up a straight line, I answered, "I make a living."

Always looking at how things can be done better, I found myself silently critiquing the nurse's presentation as she gave me instructions on how to prepare myself for the surgery and what to expect. To familiarize us all to the surroundings and to show us what a patient looks like immediately after surgery, the nurse took my family and me to the intensive care unit where I would go after surgery. As a physician, I had been there many times. Now through different eyes, I saw what a patient looked like after surgery: very weak, pale, and hooked up to tubes and a ventilator.

My rabbi visited and asked, "What do you fear most?" My immediate answer, given without thought, was, "Dying." It seemed like the right thing to say. But after a moment's reflection, I gave a more honest answer, "Coming out of this a different person—at the worst, having a stroke, but, short of that, having a different personality, losing my sense of humor." I asked him, "What's the appropriate prayer for this moment?" He replied, "the Sh'ma," a signature prayer of Judaism, which is a declaration of faith and belief in God. I had recited this prayer hundreds of times during my lifetime, but it took on new and more personal meaning to me this time when I once more repeated, "And you shall love the Lord your God with all your heart" and "These words which I command you shall be in your heart."

That evening, the nurse told me to shower and to scrub my entire body with a special soap to minimize the chance of infection after surgery. I scrubbed long and hard, anything I could do to ensure success.

The surgeon had dropped in earlier to talk and answer questions and had told me to call him at home if I had any further concerns. At 10 p.m., I called him to point out that I had athlete's foot; I had some time ago read a medical article that suggested that such a condition, even though minor, risked contamination of the vein that was to be taken from my leg as a bypass graft. Even then I was still personally involved in my care. He acknowledged my concern and assured me that he would pay special attention to the donor vein.

Finally I asked myself, "What strengths, what prior experiences could I call upon from my experience of fifty years?" I recalled my mother's life and the example of her courage and equanimity as she dealt with breast cancer. I recalled my days in college and medical school when, at a certain point in preparing for an exam, I would declare, "I've done all I can do," and I would quit studying. At about 10:30 on this night before my surgery, I said to myself, "I've done all I can do. It's time to relax. This is a new experience for me. Let's see what I can learn from it."

I felt good about myself. I felt that I had made peace with my father and my sister, with whom my relationships were at times volatile. I felt I had lived a good life. I was proud of my marriage and of where my children were in their own lives. I was at ease and as serene as I have ever been.

On Friday morning, the day of surgery, I was awakened at 5:30, and I showered and scrubbed again. My family arrived, and they accompanied me to the door of the operating room suite. This was the summer of the Iran-Contra hearings in the Congress and among my last words to them, to lighten the moment, were, "Reagan knew." An IV was started, and that's the last thing I remember before waking up after surgery.

At different times during the period of surgery, friends, the hospital director of nursing, and our rabbi visited my family as they waited at the hospital. It meant a great deal to them.

My next memory was a nurse saying to me, "Dr. X, wake up." I was connected to a ventilator, a number of tubes, and a cardiac monitor, the normal routine. My family visited, and I asked for a clipboard, pencil, and paper, on which I wrote, "Reagan knew," signaling to them, and validating for myself, that I was intellectually intact and my sense of humor was still there.

The next few days brought various treatments and manipulations. Still looking after myself, when the tube connecting me to the ventilator was to be removed, I signaled the anesthesiologist, "Be sure to deflate the cuff." I noticed blood on my leg wound dressing and asked the nurse if that was unusual. The nurse said, "More than we usually see," and that concerned me. Later that day, the surgeon told me that the amount of blood was normal. I had chills and wondered whether they were related to one of my medicines. My doctor had the same thought and discontinued the drug. In anticipation of the removal of a tube from my chest, I took a codeine pill, and that was the last of the narcotics I required for surgical pain. I coughed frequently and used the "blow bottles" to minimize the risk of lung infection. I helped to take care of myself.

On Monday, three days after surgery, I no longer needed quite so much observation and was moved to a step-down ward. That evening, I noticed sporadic irregularities of my heartbeat and then an abrupt change to a rapid heart rate. An alarm must have gone off at the nurse's desk; she appeared and told me what I already knew. She phoned the cardiologist—not mine, but the one on call—and he prescribed an intravenous drug. I said, "Call Dr. Y [my own cardiologist]," and he prescribed a different medication. I wondered if the intravenous line was running and delivering the medicine adequately. I wondered if the nurse would have called my doctor if I hadn't asked. I wondered if the nurses knew what they were doing. My heart continued to beat rapidly. One nurse told me my blood pressure was down.

I was rushed back to the intensive care unit. By now I was having pain in my arm. "Please ask Dr. Y to come in," I said to the nurse. I still had a part in overseeing my care. I felt that if I didn't stay involved, harm could occur.

My mind raced. My blood pressure is down and I'm having pain; my grafts must be closing. I could die. All of this preparation and surgery has been for nothing. My main defenses—denial, intellectualization, rationalization, and humor—no longer worked. Instead, for the first time, I felt real terror. Afraid to hear the answer, I had to ask the doctor, "Will I survive?" "Yes," he answered gently and with reassurance, and then he said, "Let go." He meant, "Relax and let us handle this." But I was still figuring, struggling, and trying to make decisions. I wondered if I could die from this, if I should ask my wife to come to the hospital for yet more last-minute words.

Now it was after midnight. Someone from the intensive care unit called my wife. Very much afraid, she struggled with whether or not to come down, felt she could not share her fears with our children or my father and sister who were staying with her, and decided to stay home. She had to deal with other feelings also, for not so long before, she had lost her mother after a long illness and years ago her father had died suddenly from heart disease. "Call as often as you want," the nurse told her. She called frequently, awake all night.

With morphine, other drugs, a blood transfusion to correct the postoperative anemia, and the passage of time, the abnormal rapid heart rhythm resolved. So did the pain. The entire episode lasted less than three hours. Nevertheless, it is the most vivid of all my memories, and when I recall those moments and retell that part of the story, I often will find myself near tears.

With the shift change at 7 a.m., a new nurse took over my care. On meeting me for the first time now, she said: "Oh! You've had heart surgery! You'll need to diet! You'll need diet foods! I sell diet foods!" I was amused by the absurdity of the situation. Here I was, having just faced what I thought was my impending death, and this nurse was talking to me about diet foods. In a less generous moment later, I thought how unaware and thoughtless this person was not to have acknowledged what the night had been like for me.

The rest of the day was uneventful, and the following day I was transferred back to the step-down ward and the same room where the arrhythmia had started. I wondered if this room was unlucky for me, but I quickly dismissed that thought with, "That's nuts! God would not be so frivolous." And then I settled down to a routine for the rest of my hospital stay.

Two nurses were primarily responsible for my care, one from 7 a.m. to 3 p.m. and another from 3 p.m. to 11 p.m. Each was competent but had a different style. One would check me over and say, "Your pulse is 80, your blood pressure is 120 over 80, your lungs are clear" in a very businesslike way. The other would do all of that, but also she would talk *with* me, inquire about my feelings, and listen. I found myself, after a few days, becoming angry with the first nurse. She never asked, "How is it going for you?" or "What's it like for you?" I weighed the pros and cons of speaking to her about this, and ultimately, a day or two before my discharge, I told her what was on my mind. I started with a compliment. "I appreciate the care you've given me," I said, and then I told her what I thought was lacking: attention to my feelings. She was defensive. "I thought that because you are a doctor, you didn't need that kind of attention," she said. "There was always someone in here visiting." (There wasn't.) I told her that the "because you are a doctor" excuse was actually a bigoted statement, for she was judging me not as an individual but as a member of a group. I was, first of all, a patient and a person, that is, a person in need, and my needs were the same as other patients'.

By the weekend, things were going well, except that I again began to notice tooth pain, similar to what I had noticed before the surgery. What did it mean? In physical therapy, I noticed some pattern changes on the EKG and asked the therapist about them. She said, "The ST segments look better." But no one had said they looked bad in the first place. More reason to worry.

On the last day, I took another stress test and passed. The uncertainty about the pain in the teeth was resolved again for the moment. Before I left the hospital, I completed a questionnaire to test how much I had learned in the cardiac rehabilitation program, which included a unit on sexual relations and at what interval after surgery I could resume. To test my knowledge, the questionnaire asked, "When can you have sex?" My answer: "October 3rd at 3:15 p.m."

I have always told patients who are returning home from a hospital stay that the first few days are difficult ones. More than one realizes, a patient depends on the hospital staff for many things, and being home without the extra hands and the reassurance of the hospital surroundings is an adjustment. And it was for me. On the first night, I had to get up several times to urinate, and each time was a major task—my wife had to help me out of bed and get me moving. I solved that problem the next day by sending my son to get a plastic urinal to keep at my bedside. I needed my wife to help me to climb stairs and to change positions, the things that nurses and others had helped with in the hospital.

Two days into my convalescence at home, I developed pain in the left side of my chest and I found that my ability to move air into the blow bottles was much less. I thought the worst: Maybe I had a pulmonary embolus, a blood clot that had injured my lung. But I didn't call my doctor and decided to wait it out. I was back looking after myself, being my own doctor. The pain resolved after a few days.

With my wife, I developed a routine—eating, walking, napping, and receiving one or two visitors a day—and that schedule took up most of the day. When friends and family visited over the next few weeks, I found that the quality of the visits and the conversation varied, from talk that was light and inconsequential to conversations that were best of all for me, the opportunity to talk about feelings and substance.

Early on August 23, my birthday, my wife received a phone call informing her that her cousin, who had been my patient and was only a few years older than I, had died suddenly of a heart-related problem. When she told me, I wept for the first time after surgery. I realized that I cried not only for him but also for myself, a release of accumulated emotion encompassing all that I had gone through over the last few weeks.

I attended a cardiac rehabilitation group three times a week. I was the youngest and the newest in the group. The therapists were optimistic and encouraging but would say to me things like, "Your blood pressure is up today. Has it been up before?" and, pointing to my heart rhythm tracing, "Are these irregular beats atrial or ventricular in origin?" I had to keep reminding them that in this place I was a patient and not the doctor.

I reflected a great deal during this time. I thought about the uncertainties of the future. Would the symptoms recur? Would my life be shortened? I recognized that I was far more robust than before the surgery. I was more active, and yet I knew there were things I could not do. It would be foolhardy, I thought, to take canoe trips into the wilderness. Though I had never done that, that limit symbolized that my illness placed restrictions on my life, which had been unrestricted before. During this time of convalescence, many symptoms came and went without explanation, but during their presence, I always asked myself, "Is this serious? Is this heart pain again?"

I found that my wife had many fears also, as she does even now. Early on, when we would walk together and I would pause for a moment, she'd ask, "Is anything wrong?" When I would come home later than expected, she worried. I learned to call if I would be late, and I still do. We had to take care of each other.

During the first few weeks after surgery, I found it easy to rationalize giving up many of my usual tasks by saying that I was "sick." My wife paid the bills and took on most of my other responsibilities. I was reluctant to give up that sick status but ultimately began to declare myself a well person, and, in mid-October, 10 weeks after the surgery, after visiting our daughter in Boston, I returned to practice for half-days. Six weeks after that, in December, I resumed full-time work.

My greatest concern on returning to work was that my mind would not be as good. But it worked as well as ever. I found that the greatest stress was the number of matters competing for my attention. When I had been home, I could concentrate on one thing at a time and take my time doing it. Now I realized that my work, medical practice, was an extremely complex logistical task, and the necessary transition to that mode of living was my greatest hurdle.

In January, my wife, daughter, and I all flew to Israel, where our son was studying, for a family reunion.

WHAT DO WE LEARN FROM THIS STORY? WHAT ARE SOME OF THE ELEMENTS OF THE HUMAN SIDE OF MEDICINE?

The details of this story provide insights into what happens when someone recognizes that he is not well, seeks advice, and connects with a physician. The patient counts on accurate diagnosis and wisely chosen therapy; what actually takes place is far more. Unless we understand how complicated the process really is, we forgo the opportunity to look at it analytically and learn from it.

To teach all of this, I use two paradigms.

The first is the *biopsychosocial model*, central to my education at the University of Rochester, where I learned to see all patients in the context of their life stories. Illness does not just happen. Important biological, psychological, and social factors—and often all three—contribute. Part of attending to patients and caring for their illnesses is discovering all the possible elements of their illnesses; neglecting any part may lead to only a partial solution and incomplete care and may delay or prevent recovery.

The second paradigm is a series of five steps, which provide a systematic approach to looking at each encounter with a patient, to learn from it, and to add to one's experience.

Step 1: the story. The patient's *story* is what really happened and the associated feelings, emotions, and reflections. It holds most of the clues to diagnosis and treatment. More than any single laboratory or x-ray test or even the physical examination of the patient, the patient's story gives broad and valuable information about what is wrong.

Step 2: the history. Inquiring about the patient's story, then editing and reshaping it into a useful oral and written format, is the process called "taking the history." The product, *the medical history*, provides the basis for defining the issues and taking action.

Step 3: the issues. By defining *the issues*, we explore all the dimensions of a medical problem and not simply the diagnosis. Issues are questions that are raised by the patient's story and the history. They include at least the following:

- What is the diagnosis? Given the diagnosis of coronary heart disease (or diabetes, appendicitis, etc.), what additional information do I need to care adequately for this patient? Unless we know all the elements of the diagnosis, we cannot completely address treatment and care.

- What are the treatment options? Of all the options, what is the best choice?

- What is the prognosis; that is, how will it turn out?

More often than not, there are additional issues, such as

- Why did this happen now?
- How will this illness progress, if treated or untreated? Will treatment make a difference?
- How will the illness affect the patient's self-image?
- How will the treatment of this illness affect the patient's other illnesses?
- What is the impact of this illness on the patient's family?
- Can the patient afford the treatment?
- Are there ethical considerations?
- What can go wrong?

Each diagnosis and problem has its own set of issues. If the story and the history are incomplete, then the definition of the issues will be inaccurate and the actions taken may be neither appropriate nor beneficial.

Step 4: the doctor-patient relationship. The *relationship* between the patient and the physician facilitates care. In each transaction, physicians should ask, "To what extent can the patient and I use that relationship to enhance care?"

Step 5: What did I learn? Step 5, the most important one in the physician's professional growth, integrates all the other steps. Asking "What did I learn?" allows insight and discovery. "What did I learn about the patient, his experience of illness and how he copes, the disease or problem, the process of obtaining the information from the patient and other sources, about what can go wrong? What did I learn about myself?" Even when an illness is incurable or when one does not get along with a patient, there is much to learn. When things go badly, it leads to asking other productive questions, "What happened? How can I prevent this from happening again?" It is the way we learn from experience.

What one learns runs the gamut from the simple to the profound. Here is what I learned from this story.

Patients consult a physician at different stages of their illness. The threshold for consulting a physician is different because each of us has different perceptions of what is going on, different fears, and different defenses. This patient used denial frequently during the early stages of his symptoms, though, as a physician, he should have known better. Other factors pertain. Timing (his children were going away) and the influence of others ("My wife made me make this appointment" is a common statement) often breach the threshold for consulting a physician.

The medical history and the story from which it is derived are important. Despite his having serious underlying heart disease, this patient had a completely normal physical exam. Only the patient's story gave the clues to the diagnosis.

For each problem, there are implied questions: What is the cause of this problem (the diagnosis)? What is the solution (the treatment)? How is it going to turn out (the prognosis)? These are some of the "technical" issues of medicine, and the physician must address each of them with each transaction.

Even with excellent care, things can go wrong. This patient experienced drug-induced chills and a disorder of heart rhythm. The physicians and nurses promptly recognized and treated each complication of treatment. Drug- and treatment-induced illnesses occur frequently.

Illness has symbolic meaning to patients, and patients have psychological reactions to illness. This patient initially felt sadness, shame, and embarrassment. Other patients may feel anger, resentment, disappointment, inadequacy, or failure. They may feel that they are being punished for previous missteps. Some see illness as an opportunity for growth. Some feel that their religion has failed them. Some feel isolated. Recognizing the diversity of meanings and psychological reactions enables the physician to individualize care.

Patients have psychological defenses, some healthy and some not so healthy. This patient's defenses included the following:

- Denial. "It's not my heart," he said when he first started having the discomfort, and he tried to reinforce this denial by climbing stairs despite the pain and by pressing on with his vacation plans.

- Intellectualization. "This is a new experience for me. Let's see what I can learn from it." He saw himself as a participant-observer. From the beginning, he critiqued the instruction and care he received and how his physicians and others said things to him. It was a new adventure.

- Humor. His comments to the admitting clerk and to his family on the way to surgery helped him and his family through the crisis, and his family shared his humor.

- Optimism. He had a sense of the future. The surgery was not an end in itself but a bridge from poorer health to better health.

- A desire to maintain some sense of control over his care. Though he did not need to call all the shots, he found himself participating actively in his care. But this was a double-edged sword. On the one hand, he would have preferred to let others care for him. As a physician, though, he was well informed about the nature of his illness and treatment and the potential complications of both, and he had expert knowledge about himself. He also knew that sometimes hospital systems fail, and so he could not stay uninvolved. This is an experience common to many who are health professionals.

Ultimately, his healthy defenses broke down and gave way to fear.

Patients have other strengths that serve them well during the stress of the illness. The task of the physician is to identify and accommodate those strengths and to encourage patients and their families to recognize and use them during their illness. Physicians need to ask, "Does the patient have the support of family, friends, a religion or faith or philosophy of life? Can these be resources for him during a period of stress?"

Religion and his synagogue community were resources for the patient in the opening story. He was aware of the ways of looking at things that his religion offered and had a relationship with his rabbi. He was able to draw upon these resources for comfort and for support. For others, religion may not be of use.

Illness is a family affair. His wife, son and daughter, and father and sister were all involved. His illness and the various steps in his recovery touched each of them in different ways. Not only did the patient have to deal with his illness, he had to deal with its impact on them. To be a complete physician, one must identify the important relationships and the important issues with each.

Others experience the drama of a patient's illness. To varying degrees, many were touched by the drama of his illness: his friends, physician-partner, office staff, patients, and rabbi. With the drama of a potentially serious illness comes redefinition and clarification of relationships. He found valued relationships that he did not know he had and disappointments in existing ones.

Previous experiences affect how patients and their families deal with the current drama. This was a crisis for the patient, but not his biggest, he reflected, and he could call upon the experience gained from other dramas in his life—his mother's illness, for example—and apply those lessons to his current drama.

His wife's father had died suddenly from a heart-related event, and now her husband's illness was a reminder of that tragedy. Nonetheless, she dealt with the current situation with equanimity. For her husband and their children, she was a stabilizing influence. Their children felt no obvious panic. They were able to talk about their own feelings and even to ask their father about his. This shared experience will serve the family well in the future, for they will remember that they weathered a severe stress together and that they can depend on each other.

Patients and their families can handle bad news. The news was overpowering at first, but they dealt with it. Physicians need not hesitate to talk about serious issues.

Illness is a stress superimposed on the patient's ongoing drama of life. Though many patients have a well adjusted and ordered life, some come to the moment of illness or surgery from a disorganized and chaotic life. If our lives are in order, we can better handle the stress of illness. As physicians, we need to be aware of what is going on in the patient's life by asking what few asked of this patient, "What's this like for you?" Is this simply heart surgery, or is this heart surgery superimposed upon, for example, a disrupted marriage, loss of income, or loss of prestige?

The drama of one's life continues despite the illness. As physicians, we write a one-word order at the end of a hospitalization: "Discharge." It would be far better if physicians were sufficiently informed about a patient to write: "Discharge to a peaceful home and family" or "Discharge to a disrupted, chaotic home." Then we might have second thoughts about the best moment to send the patient home.

Serious illness is chaotic. Illness is not as simple as "I got sick and then I got better," but rather a series of ups and downs, surprises, catastrophes and rescues, and human reactions—some great and some disappointing—from patients, families, physicians, and other professionals. Physicians can acknowledge the chaos to patients. At the very least, they should not contribute to it with ill-chosen words, actions uncoordinated with other colleagues, or inaccessibility.

Illness, serious or not, is laden with uncertainty. Patients, their families, and physicians need to deal with that uncertainty. When we acknowledge uncertainty, we often reduce anxiety. To this day, the patient believes that the reason he required so little medicine for pain after the surgery was that he was well informed about what to expect. In each illness, a statement about prognosis recognizes and addresses uncertainty.

There are no barriers in the hospital. Certainly, physical barriers cease to exist. Hospital staff enter a room without knocking, and frequent interruptions punctuate each hour. There are no emotional barriers either. Ill patients are vulnerable physically and psychologically. Emotions and feelings are bared. But the barrier is down the other way also, for this is an opportunity for a sensitive physician to help address fears and faulty relationships that may hamper recovery and a successful outcome. Serious illness is an opportunity for patients to explore their values and philosophies of life, to validate themselves, and to heal relationships.

Language and how physicians and other health professionals communicate have great impact on patients and their families, who hang on every word from physicians and others associated with their care. "The blood on your dressing is more than we usually see" were words of small consequence to the nurse, but such comments raised additional questions of uncertainty for the patient. Interpretation should accompany every piece of information. Compassion, understanding, and accessibility comfort and help prevent panic.

There are bigotry and prejudice in the medical setting. Most of this is due to thoughtlessness. Bigotry or prejudice means viewing a person too narrowly or as a member of a group—for example, an ethnic minority, immigrants, the elderly, women, "heart patients," physicians—rather than as an individual. When challenged about the neglect of his feelings as a patient, the nurse squandered the opportunity to address the fears, apprehensions, and sense of uncertainty that the physician-patient had in common with other patients. As physicians we need to cross the barrier from a one-dimensional view of patients to a fuller view. Prejudice limits accurate, creative decision making.

Medicine is a collaborative profession. Often, more than one person is involved in the care of an illness. Each needs to know how to work with the others and with the patient. There is always someone who does not get the message.

Being there is important. The contemporary actor and director Woody Allen said that "80 percent of life is 'showing up.'"[1] Being there in person, rather than calling or delegating, carries extra weight with the patient. Though the telephoned instructions to the nurse during the patient's frightening period of the arrhythmia might well have been appropriate, the cardiologist's *presence* provided the recognition of the seriousness and the reassurance that the patient needed.

Illness is a drama, and the patient is the center of the drama. Neither the physician nor the hospital nor the third parties—hospital, corporate structure, insurance company—takes precedence over what is in the best interest of the patient.

The story is never over. A hospital encounter or a visit to the office may last only fifteen minutes, but the story goes on seven days a week, twenty-four hours a day. Even when it seems as if the drama is completed, there are always more chapters. There is always something more to do in refining the diagnosis, treatment, or prognosis or supporting the patient and the family.

Stories teach. Wise physicians read between the lines of a brief history like the one at the beginning of this chapter. They look beyond diagnosis and treatment to see that in each illness, there is a drama that encompasses almost all the elements we learned about in understanding this patient's story. Then they draw on their experience in order to provide complete care, technically excellent and complete on the human side.

To develop the medical history, one needs the story. To see illness in the context of the person, one needs the story. To see an ill person in the context of the whole person, one needs the story. When the diagnosis seems elusive, when there are different points of view among consultants, or when they want to find out how a patient is coping, wise physicians will return to the patient's story.

Reflecting on this patient's story and asking, "What did I learn?" allows us to define many of the elements of the human side of medicine. Each of the subsequent sections addresses them in more detail as we discover what it is like to be a patient and what it is like to be a physician. We will start with short histories from moments at the end of patients' lives when technical matters are less crucial than human ones.

Chapter 2

Learning from End-of-Life Stories

"Preferring a discussion of parts failing to persons dying."

Moments exist in medicine where the need for the human side dwarfs the need for technology and a statement that "things have gotten a lot worse in the last week" has more meaning than "the kidney function is worse today." When patients, families, and physicians recognize that life is coming to an end, they fashion their decisions differently, often cease measures to support life, and concentrate on comfort. Together they often decide in advance not only what they should not do, but what will help. Reflecting on the meaning of these moments enhances our understanding of what is the essence of medical care for *all* patients and their families.

The comedian lay dying, the story goes, and his pals gathered at his bedside, where one of them said, "It must be tough to die." His response: "Dying is easy. *Comedy* is difficult." Dying may not be so easy, but we need to ask these questions: Do physicians make dying more difficult than it has to be? Do they prolong treatment inappropriately? Do they squander opportunities to intervene effectively? What can we learn, as we answer these questions, that has universal application to caring for all who are ill? From my practice, here are four stories that help to define and clarify the issues.

TALKING ABOUT SERIOUS MATTERS WITH PATIENTS

Case 1: A Middle-Aged Man with Widespread Cancer

In his mid-50s, a successful executive had incurable cancer of the kidney with lung metastases, for which chemotherapy was not very effective. He was hospitalized because of vomiting, which was improving with intravenous fluids and medicines to control his nausea. His urologist asked me to see him for "general medical evaluation" and help with his long-term care.

At our first meeting, the patient told me he was aware of his poor prognosis, had spoken in depth with his wife and children about it, and had already made his own funeral arrangements. He seemed very much at ease. I saw him daily, and our conversations were substantial as we talked not only about his illness but also about his life, his career, his relationship with his wife and children, his philosophy of life, and his values.

Here is what I learned:

One can talk about serious matters with patients. In this and all of the other stories in this chapter, my role was not difficult. While I needed to choose my words carefully, the honesty of the conversation and the depth of the discussion of facts and feelings became the foundation for our further decisions. Our trust in each other contributed to the effectiveness of the therapy. Physicians need not shrink from being straightforward, "preferring a discussion of parts failing to persons dying."[1]

The patient may see silence on these matters as the equivalent of a lie, and caught in a lie, a physician may have to work very hard to reestablish trust. Hardly ever is this the first crisis the patient has faced. When we fail to speak honestly, we assume the patient cannot handle the information. Experience shows otherwise. My discussions with this patient provided me the opportunity to discover his strengths, validate them as a resource for him, and shore up his weaknesses.

Caring for a dying patient can be an especially rich time for the physician. I looked forward to seeing this patient each day in the hospital. I went from learning *about* him to learning *from* him. He started as my patient and became my teacher.

ALLOWING THE PATIENT TO EXPRESS HER VIEWS, AND EXPLORING HER VALUES

Case 2: A 60-Year-Old Woman with a Pancreatic Tumor

The gastroenterologist asked me to see this 60-year-old woman with pancreatic cancer for help in managing her diabetes. She had developed jaundice, which indicated bile duct obstruction. After abdominal surgery showed incurable cancer, tubes fed her intravenously and drained her stomach, abdominal incision, and bladder. Each day she needed four insulin injections. The gastroenterologist and the surgeon were managing her case, each taking care of only part of her. She had no primary physician and no close family.

I reviewed her hospital chart, interviewed and examined her, and made recommendations regarding the management of the diabetes—not a difficult task. In addition, I wondered if anyone had asked her, "What's this like for you? How do you feel about going on with the treatment?" So I asked. The experience was overwhelming, she said, a nightmare. Given the seriousness of the diagnosis and the hopelessness of the outcome, she would prefer that treatment cease; all she wanted was comfort. She was relieved that I asked. It had not occurred to her to voice her views to the other physicians, nor had they given her the opportunity.

Here is what I learned:

Patients need to be authorized to voice their views. Often they do not because they have never been in the habit of doing so in any situation, medical or otherwise; because they are intimidated by professionals; because they are afraid they will be viewed as "giving up"; or simply because they do not know that it is allowed. While people are more vulnerable when they are ill, they are also more accessible to inquiries from physicians, nurses, social workers, and clergy about their feelings, values, and philosophy of life. We should take advantage of that accessibility.

The physician needs to explore the patient's values. Failing that, one may inadvertently provide unwanted care or find unexplained conflict with the patient's wishes.

There is more to comfort than pain control. Even when it seems we can do no more, we can do a great deal. Many formal religious prayers for the ill call for "healing of the spirit" along with "healing of the body." Even if someone's body cannot be healed, there is still the opportunity to find comfort in resolving conflicts and healing relationships. Part of our responsibility as members of the healing professions is to facilitate that process. Treatment includes many actions other than those that cure, and there is much that a physician can do to provide comfort and guidance for the patient and the family. Without this critical activity, the illness becomes unnecessarily chaotic, the patient and the family may feel isolated or abandoned, and they may squander precious time.

THE EVER-CHANGING ROLE OF THE PHYSICIAN

Case 3: A 70-Year-Old Man with Widespread Cancer

On his return from a well-known medical center where this patient had been receiving chemotherapy for widespread cancer, the retired executive's wife called to ask that I become his physician. The initial treatment had failed, an experimental drug was being offered with "less than 25 percent chance of success," and he was having ongoing pain that medicine poorly controlled. Stopping chemotherapy had not been considered. The adult children lived at least three hours away by plane. Prior to this call, he had no primary physician in his hometown.

On my first visit to his home, we concentrated on pain control, and I prescribed ibuprofen, a mild but often effective drug when given regularly several times a day. Subsequent visits concentrated on achieving better pain control using morphine, on helping him understand his illness (he knew that the prognosis was poor), and on addressing alternative ways of treating the progressive malignancy, including more chemotherapy. He declined the latter.

With his wife, we also talked about their experience and their fears. "What's this been like for you?" I asked. It was clear that they had a strong, mutually supportive relationship and that they were sharing the story of the drama of his illness with their out-of-town children, who began to appear at their home for prolonged stays. As time went on, a hospice nurse became involved, and she and I collaborated with the family on his care. Even though his condition continued to decline, the family was becoming more and more self-sufficient in meeting his needs and their own. With their concurrence, my visits became more widely spaced; they did not need me as much. He died within a few months of my first visit.

Here is what I learned:

Once more, *medicine is a collaborative effort, and the most important participants in the collaboration are the patient and family.* Consulting physicians, social workers, nurses, and clergy help. Their different points of view may reflect their professional paradigms of care, who they are as individuals, and their values and prejudices, which they may not even recognize. But there must always be a *primary* caregiver, the general contractor who is ultimately responsible and who can integrate diverse points of view into a single set of recommendations and a plan. Someone has to be in charge. Though I provided no specific anticancer treatment, I did much more. I assessed his needs and the needs of his family in the broadest sense, and I addressed his prognosis with all of them. I involved others—family and hospice nurse—in his care.

Illness is not a single moment but a dynamic process in which people can come to terms, make peace, and learn how to cope. The physician's role needs to be dynamic to accommodate these changes. Though I was more important to the patient and his family in the beginning, as the family rallied, became more active in his care and in looking after each other, and as other professionals became involved, the need for a physician lessened. To have continued frequent visits might have been seen as an intrusion.

DISCOVERING WHERE THE PATIENT IS

Case 4: End-Stage Heart Disease in a 70-Year-Old Woman

Twenty years after her first myocardial infarct (heart attack) this 70-year-old college professor was having more and more difficulty with her heart: repeated episodes of congestive heart failure and moments of sudden prolonged rapid heartbeat requiring an implanted defibrillator. Usually their recurrence was unpredictable, and so they were all the more distressing for her and her family. After one of these events, while she was still unconscious, I called her husband and daughters together to talk about the poor prognosis. They declined the opportunity to declare, "Do not resuscitate," and they became angry that I had even opened the subject. The patient again recovered, and two years passed, during which several more episodes occurred and her health continued to decline. During this time, I often asked her alone or together with her husband, "How are things overall for you? What's all this like for you?" She was displeased whenever I included her husband in the conversations, and at her last visit declared, "I'm changing doctors! Coming to see you is like sitting *shiva* [i.e., coming to a Jewish house of mourning]." She died a few months later.

Here is what I learned:

Sometimes, even with the best and most sensitive of intentions, things run amok in the physician-patient relationship. If there is no recognition of the patient's and the family's expectations, there can be no real alliance between them and the physician. Physicians need to discover how *the patient* sees her illness, what *her* concept of the cause is, what issues *she* sees, what *her* view of the prognosis is, what *she* sees as the impact on her family and *her* resources, and what *she* fears. Those may be fear of unrelenting pain, emotional isolation from family, or abandonment by the physician. Unless we start where the patient and the family are, we risk undermining the relationship and magnifying the panic that can come with having a serious illness.

Be realistic, but do not remove all hope. Tailor the message to the needs of the individual. In this case, removing hope when the patient and her family were not ready for that step was premature.

SEEING BEYOND THE OBVIOUS DETAILS

Regardless of what we know about a certain illness or a certain patient, there is always more to learn. As physicians, we enlarge our knowledge and our effectiveness by learning from patients. That is truly learning from experience.

However complex the data, however many consultants are involved, the patients' experience of illness, their feelings, and their values help to fashion a plan of care and enhance its effectiveness and appropriateness. Especially when time is precious, we can squander time if the care is not what the patient wants. When there is conflict between the patient and family members, we need to find out where each is and how each sees the illness and the situation. Sometimes clergy or social workers can help reach consensus by clarifying the issues.

To gain access to these issues, I ask the patient such open-ended questions as "What's this like for you?" "What bothers you the most?" or even simply, "What do you want?"

To address end-of-life decisions before the moment of urgency strikes, I say, "I hope you know by now that we can talk about anything. By that I mean, if you don't understand what I have said to you or if you disagree with what I have recommended, you can feel comfortable saying that to me, and we can discuss it." This statement provides the context for me to say next, "I could conceive of a situation where we might *not* be able to discuss it. Either you would be so ill that you might be unable to comprehend or you might be unconscious, and I would not want to do anything that you wouldn't want me to do. For instance, if your heart would stop beating or if you would require machinery to keep you going, what would you want me to do?" If the patient is unable to be part of such a decision, I ask the same of the responsible person, substituting: "If your mother [or daughter, etc.] were able to speak for herself, what do you think she would want us to do?" That is far better than "What do you think we should do?" a question that places too great a burden on the surrogate.

For patients with illnesses in which the prospect of pain may be a substantial concern, I address that issue specifically, if they have not, and assure them that "whatever pain you have can be managed and minimized." I indicate that "I will not abandon you" by words and staying involved. I always give them a new appointment to see or call me.

I ask, "Who are your resources? Who is your community? To what extent is your religion or faith or philosophy of life a resource to you?"

If I am asked, "How much time do I have?" I answer the best way I know how. Not "three weeks" or "three to six months," but rather, "I don't know of any way to answer that question precisely. But you must know with this sort of illness that there are many uncertainties and that time is precious." I believe that the question is often not one of numerical inquiry but rather a request for a discussion of prognosis. It is another opportunity to begin—or continue—a conversation about their understanding of the illness, fears, resources, relationships, expectations, and values.

I write letters of sympathy to survivors, and always, when appropriate, I include the statement, "You did all you possibly could." I know that such losses are often followed by feelings of guilt: "If only I had recognized the significance of his chest pain. If only I had told him once more how much I cared."

Though these case histories are about people with terminal illnesses, each provides insights into ways in which physicians can attend to the human side of medicine for every patient. The lessons are universal. None involves complex technology. Good physicians see beyond the most obvious details. Each sentence in the story is but a "headline," a clue to what is really going on and what it is like for the patient and the family. Skilled physicians use their experience to inquire more completely and to provide more definitive care. For all of this, we need time, and the next chapter addresses that dimension of medicine.

Chapter 3

Time

"It does not take an excessive amount of time to be a compassionate physician."

Patients need time. Among the highest compliments a patient can give to a physician is: "You always seem to have time for me. When I'm with you, it seems like you have nobody else on your mind." One of the most frequent complaints is: "My doctor doesn't take time. He's always got one foot out the door." Physicians need time also. Really good doctors say, "I always have time for you" or "I'll take all the time I need." Compromising on time compromises the quality of the diagnosis, treatment, prognosis, and relationship.

Especially troubling are patients'—and students'—statements, almost as if they were established truth, that "managed care dictates that doctors can spend no more than ten minutes (sometimes it's five) with each patient." It is an untenable position and an invalid observation. Dollar for dollar, time is less expensive than most tests, procedures, equipment, and drugs. Fifteen minutes of a physician's time costs far less than an MRI and can be far more productive.

PATIENTS AND THEIR FAMILIES NEED TIME

Patients and their families need time to understand and be understood, to absorb, adjust, cope, accept, make changes, and heal physically and spiritually.

It takes time to tell the story. An undergraduate wrote: "It feels very frightening to think that a doctor can confuse a patient's diagnosis because he or she doesn't have time to listen. . . . Perhaps telling stories was the only time where I felt I was in control."

It takes time for the patient to find meaning in the illness. A chaplain described this as "a gentle process, something that cannot be forced. It requires guiding with questions."[1]

It takes time to deal with a difficult child, parent, or dilemma, to adjust to an illness, and to accept advice. We cannot always expect an immediate change in an opinion or behavior. We cannot, overnight, cope with the impact of a diagnosis of cancer, heart disease, or other chronic illness. Nor can we decide quickly about having major surgery, undergoing chemotherapy, or declining treatment. It takes time to come to grips with a need to change our style of living—eating or work habits or a nicotine addiction. Patients and families think things over between visits to the physician, think about their physician's advice, ruminate, and talk things over with others. What goes on behind the scenes is substantial. They do "homework"; they read, they search the Internet, they may even get another medical opinion on their own.

It takes time for the patient to make peace with a spouse, a friend, or an estranged relative. Time, however limited, allows unfinished business to take place—the healing of a relationship or the resolution of some long-standing conflict.

It takes time to say good-bye. One student wrote about her dog's final months with cancer. "Medicine gave me time to say good-bye—not overnight, but over a period of eight months [after the diagnosis was made]. I will always be thankful for the extra time I had with her . . . for I learned to truly appreciate her and all she gave to my life."

PHYSICIANS NEED TIME

It takes time to establish a relationship and to get to truly know the patient. "Each case has its own natural life," my wife, the social worker, taught me. It has its own period: the time in which the story develops, the relationship matures, the illness proceeds, the needs become clear, and the opportunities become obvious. To this I add, "And the story is never over." Often something new happens or a new insight occurs to the patient or to the physician that allows the drama to make progress. The story goes on. And so we must allow time to elapse and not inappropriately hurry the process.

It takes time to listen to a patient's story, fashion it into a coherent history, think about it, clarify it, ponder a diagnosis, look at various ways to integrate the problems, track the course of treatment, consider the significance of the response or lack of response to treatment, and explain it all to the patient and family. I like to wake people up with this story: "The office administrator of a group of cardiac surgeons called them together for a discussion of their financial status. 'Our income is down in the last year. From now on, you need to do each cardiac bypass operation in one and a half hours instead of three.'" "How many of you would like to go to that office?" I ask. No more should a heart surgeon be asked to shorten inappropriately the time it takes to do bypass surgery than should any physician be asked to compromise on the time spent with a patient in these other activities.

It takes time to examine the patient's values. When I spoke with a woman about her disease, incurable cancer of the esophagus, I told her, "This is not only a technical issue, but also a philosophical and spiritual one." Then we could explore her values and agree upon the best mode of care compatible with her philosophy of life, and she could plan how to use her remaining days.

It takes time to explain in depth, to "reason out loud," and to address all of the patient's questions. Some patients have many questions, not necessarily because they are distrustful, compulsive, or poorly educated, but because they may be more informed than the physician realizes, or apprehensive about their health. A first-year medical student observed, "It does not take a long time to tell the truth, just as it does not take an excessive amount of time to be a compassionate physician."

It takes time to negotiate, to find an accommodation, to come to an understanding, to define a common goal, and to appreciate what it is like to be the patient. In the midst of any complex illness, it takes time to review the entire course of the illness, to help patients recognize their strengths, to acknowledge the uncertainties, offer hope, and assure them of the physician's commitment to them. We cannot address all these issues in a brief time, nor can a few short conversations explore in depth the issues the patient and the physician need to deal with.

It takes time to collaborate, to identify, clarify, and validate the issues for all the participants. Developing a strategy for care and altering it when appropriate take time.

It takes time to reflect on simple and complex illnesses and patients and to react to those reflections. Time allows us to learn from each transaction and to integrate what we have learned into our experience. We need time to step back and say, "This was a great day [or an awful one]. What's this all about? What did I learn? What did I learn that's more universally applicable?" Time facilitates reflection.

Dealing with the human side of medicine involves an extra commitment in time. It may involve some compromise of income. Yet it is all a matter of values. The quality of the transaction depends not only on the outcome, but also on the process and the relationship. If all of this depends on time, then physicians, most of all, cannot compromise on time.

It is time well spent. And it is part of the joy of medicine.

Chapter 4

Learning from Patients' Experiences

"When I have a physician who listens, it's magic."

Being a patient goes beyond the symptoms of the illness to the *experience* of being ill. Anatole Broyard wrote, "Each man is ill in his own way."[1] He reflected on his illness, metastatic cancer of the prostate: "My friends flatter me by calling my performance courageous or gallant, but my doctor should know better. He should be able to imagine the aloneness of the critically ill."[2]

Consciously or not, patients apply their philosophy of life to the medical situation at hand. Common sense is often at the foundation. An 80-year-old man reflected on his illness, unstable angina, which was improving with medication. "I know it's better, but I'm 75 years old. . . . It's like, 'We've got a good car, but it's twelve years old, so shall we drive [from St. Paul] to Los Angeles?' I don't need to take unnecessary chances." Our philosophy of life affects difficult decisions about tests and treatments including transfusions, surgery, chemotherapy, and end-of-life care. Part of the physician's task is to discover each patient's philosophy and needs. Sometimes the doctor has to read between the lines.

Not from any textbook or formal teaching, but from patients, their families, and other sources, I learned all of what follows.

Patients need moral support. "You have a 90 percent chance of improvement with this surgery" is information. "We'll do everything we can to make this turn out well" is support.

Patients need to be understood. A nursing home resident who had long-standing unexplained abdominal pain said, "Thank you for spending the time with me. It doesn't solve anything, but I appreciate the fact that you try to understand me." Another patient told me, "If you find a doctor who understands you, you can do anything."

Patients need to be validated. "One must visit a wise man from time to time to discover what one already knows."[3] Patients may already have figured out that their symptoms are not serious, but they need the reassurance from someone with a credential, the "wise man" called "Doctor." A patient may be grieving over the loss of a spouse and need to be reassured by his physician that he is not going crazy. Even though a patient may be expert in the care of her diabetes, she still needs reassurance that she is doing the right thing. "You didn't minimize," one patient told me. "You believed in me," said another.

Patients need to understand. The patient and family may be hearing things for the first time and need the perspective and the time to understand what the physician, who has been wrestling with the dilemma for a while, already comprehends. The patient, members of the family, and the physician each may have a different view. Not recognizing this phenomenon may explain why there is conflict among them. Only when each of the participants—physician, patient, and family—is dealing with the same information in the same context can they be allies. Often it is not so much the degree of severity of the symptom that brings the patient to the doctor as the need for explanation.

When a 49-year-old man developed chest pain after seven days of treatment for pneumonia, he thought, "I'm back to square one. This is the pain I had in the beginning of my illness. The treatment has failed." The physician knew better. The pain was pleurisy, caused by friction between the injured surface of the healing lung and the inner chest wall. By explaining this to the patient, he was able to reassure him. All the patient needed was adequate explanation. He was less bothered by the pain than by the questions: "What does it mean? How will it turn out?"

Patients need to talk to the physician; sometimes a surrogate just will not do. When a 40-year-old woman with rheumatoid arthritis had more aching in her hands and wrists, she called the doctor. The office assistant took the message and relayed these instructions from the doctor to the patient: Use heat and acetaminophen. The patient needed to talk with the doctor, to explain her symptoms, and to talk about her concerns and her fears. She wanted his attention and reassurance. Only a direct conversation could meet those needs.

Patients need context. When a radiologist told my patient that "you have many small changes on the brain MRI," he and his wife called me in panic, concerned that this was the beginning of Alzheimer's disease. I was able to provide context and reassurance that the changes were not significant.

However serious or trivial the illness or complaint, patients need a prognosis, a prediction of how it is going to turn out. Otherwise fantasies may take over. "There's a better than 90 percent chance that this therapy will cure your lymphoma, though we'll keep track of it for years to come." "Your sore throat should be better after a few days." "Within six weeks of therapy, your shoulder will be back to normal." After such an explanation, a patient told me, "If you know how it's going to turn out, that it's going to get better, you can handle a lot more." When my 65-year-old patient told me about the numbness on the side of his toe, a minor annoyance, he did not need an explanation of the cause and certainly not a description of the nerve anatomy of the foot. All he wanted was reassurance that it was not anything serious.

Patients have unasked questions and undeclared fears that need to be identified and explored. I ask, "What about this illness worries you the most?" Here are four vignettes.

- In her mid-20s, a social worker, the wife of a physician-in-training, developed a severe sore throat and swollen lymph nodes in her neck. She was concerned that she might have leukemia and was relieved when her physician, not her husband, told her, "You have mononucleosis."
- In her late-20s, a newly married junior executive developed painful urination. Her doctor treated her for a bladder infection. When the pain persisted and she noticed blood in her urine after a day of treatment, she called the physician, not because of the pain, but only to be reassured that she did not have a serious illness.
- A 35-year-old bookkeeper who was tired and breathless was relieved to learn that she had Grave's disease, an overactive thyroid gland. Her sister had developed heart disease at a young age, and this was her real worry.
- Though he had known about his hypertension for five years, a 45-year-old man finally consulted a physician. He feared that he might be at risk for stroke after he learned of his friend's stroke.

Patients need consistency. More than one explanation from different sources is confusing and adds to the chaos of a serious illness. Patients want an integrated story and consistent explanation and advice. A 70-year-old man with an abnormal heart valve, now infected, was faced with this di-

lemma. The cardiologist told him that he should continue to take anticoagulant medicine to prevent a stroke. The hematologist told him that
anticoagulant medicine could lead to brain hemorrhage. It was up to his
primary care physician to integrate this disparate advice into a single recommendation. Indeed, in situations where many specialists are involved,
this may be the most important function of the primary doctor.

Sometimes patients need physicians just to listen. When her elderly mother
complains to her about her problems, my friend asks, "Are you telling me
this because you want advice, or because you want me to listen?" Sometimes the patient needs neither answer nor remedy but simply someone to
listen with respect and without interruption. A patient told me, "To have
someone who listens and gives thoughtful, trustworthy advice is a blessing.
When I have a physician who listens, it's magic."

Patients need a sense that the doctor cares. Clergy speak of "the ministry of
presence." A medical student called it "listening with your eyes"; that is,
paying attention, *attending*. While camping, a 40-year-old real estate agent
suffered third-degree leg burns when his stove exploded. He had already
seen two physicians when he called me with concern about the adequacy of
his care. I arranged for a burn specialist to see him and reviewed with the
specialist my patient's history of inflammatory bowel disease and treatment. Thereafter I was not directly involved in his care, which took place
at another hospital. The patient thanked me "for orchestrating." "But I did
no more than you do in your work," I said, for all I had done was facilitate
the connection. "But you did it with love," he responded. Doing it "with
love" may be an overstatement, but being pro-active and involved certifies
the physician's commitment.

The house call is presence amplified. At home, physicians can see how
patients and their families interact and adjust to an illness, how they maintain their home, and how self-sufficient they are. The home is a personal essay about memories, relationships, possessions, and values. Physicians who
practice in small towns and are part of the community may already know
much of this about their patients; in a city practice, the house call provides
some of those insights. Especially if patients are inarticulate, seeing them at
home tells a lot. These days, when a house call is rare, it is an impressive
gesture to the patient and family. Years later, patients still refer with fond-
ness and appreciation to "the time you came to our home."

Patients need an advocate. Being an advocate and a general contractor who
coordinates care is an important role for doctors. My son, not a doctor, tells of
his volunteer work with the homeless in New York City. "Sometimes they
would need to go to ten different agencies to get all that they needed. If they
could actually do all of that, they could run their lives." Patients need physi-

cian-advocates to direct them through the complex system of care. If they could do all of that alone, they would not need a doctor. Broyard writes, "The doctor is the patient's only family in a foreign country."[4]

Some patients may be reluctant to call their physician. An 80-year-old friend had been vomiting for three days and finally called me rather than call her personal physician after office hours. I examined her at home, found that she was dehydrated and still unable to eat, admitted her to the hospital, and began treatment. I notified her doctor the following morning. Defensive and angry because she had not called him, the doctor failed to recognize the variety of reasons that patients do not call immediately: because they are afraid of a serious diagnosis, they fear hospitalization and uncomfortable tests, they may be embarrassed by their symptoms, it is human to hope that a symptom or an illness will go away, or they do not want to bother the doctor. Sometimes it is because the doctor is not that easy to contact. Patients have their own way of making decisions, and these patterns may reflect the quality of their experiences with other physicians. Some move quickly to settle unanswered questions, and others delay. Some need immediate answers; others are comfortable waiting. Physicians need to accommodate these differences.

Some patients may be embarrassed by the presence of their illness, its duration, or its lack of improvement. A cascade of complications befell my 45-year-old patient after a work accident, and she was seeing many physicians—and an attorney—over a period of years. Some of the doctors were sympathetic, and others were skeptical and often failed to pay attention to her symptoms. When she first saw me, she was embarrassed to tell her story to yet another doctor. Her wise attorney observed, "She may be complex, but she is no less entitled."

Some patients are embarrassed by being on a medical assistance program, which makes them feel even more dependent. On that subject, my 40-year-old patient with diabetes and hypertension commented, "It's sort of like having a sheet that's a little too small on a cold night. If you pull it up over your shoulders, your feet get cold. If you pull it down, your shoulders get cold."

Some patients fear being dependent on family members and friends or on a physician who may underestimate the seriousness of their illness. A patient with cancer of the pancreas told me, "You don't get top-notch care unless the doctors think you're top-notch sick."

Some patients fear being too narrowly defined as a sick person. Long ago I stopped referring to patients as "diabetics"; instead, each is "a person with diabetes." I am careful to make that point directly to the patient when I say, "Your diabetes does not define you."

Patients need to feel safe anywhere in the system. Whether patients are ill in the hospital, a nursing home, the physician's office, or at home, they need to feel that there is a plan of care, access to someone in charge, and attention to all their needs.

What do we learn from all of this? Physicians need to find out what it is like for the patient and ask, "How does this patient handle crisis? How is he handling *this* crisis?" Self-reflection does not hurt. The physician can ask, "What would this be like for me if I were in the same situation?" It helps when physicians examine their personal experiences with illness. One of my goals in teaching students is to help them learn from their and their families' experiences. These lessons provide a context for examining further what it is like to be a patient. The next chapter recounts some of the students' stories.

Chapter 5

Learning from Students' Experiences

"After all, I know the pain best."

Many physicians relate stories from their youth with a common theme: There was a serious or dramatic illness in their family, sometimes their own illness, and a good or bad outcome or experience with the medical care. They were *involved* in the drama; it had its effect on them and their lives. Part of who we are as physicians is a reflection of our experiences.

Many physicians had good role models, impressive people who had special skills, "a nice bedside manner," performed what seemed like a dramatic rescue from a serious illness, or simply developed a relationship with the physicians-to-be, often long before they ever thought about a career. Some models may have been bad ones, moving the prospective physician to declare, "When I become a doctor, I will do it better." Everyone who becomes a physician has experiences upon which to draw in order to become a good doctor. From the human standpoint, students may be at their best when they are involved not as physicians-in-training but rather as patients or family members, relating at the level of their most genuine feelings and untainted by the jargon and patterns of medical thinking.

Here's the proof. To provide beginning data for the "Seminar in the Human Side of Medicine" at Macalester College, I give my students this written assignment:

1. Tell the story of an illness that you or a family member experienced.
2. How did you or the family member handle it? What was it like for you or the family member or all of you? What was the best part? What was the worst part?
3. *What do you learn* from your reflections?

I am always struck by the variety of illnesses the students have experienced and the depth of their reflections. Among the illnesses they have personally had are diabetes, hyperthyroidism, traumatic rupture of a kidney, ulcerative colitis, Crohn's disease (an inflammatory disease of the intestine, also called ileitis), depression, Hodgkin's disease (a malignancy), seizures, Bell's palsy (paralysis of a facial nerve), and appendicitis. Their family members have had strokes, heart disease, pneumonia, emphysema, and cancer. One student even told of her dog's malignancy and its impact on her and her family.

Most have received fine care, but some have faced erroneous diagnoses, prejudice, despair and desperation, loneliness, hopelessness, helplessness, and thoughtless professionals. From their experience, they have learned that so much important information about patients and their families is overlooked, that there are universal qualities to illness, that people have different strengths and ways of dealing with a crisis or dilemma, that illness is a family affair, and that uncertainties surround most illnesses. Here are some of their insights.

Of her illness, Crohn's disease, a junior wrote of complex feelings and her disappointment with some of her physicians' actions.

At 14, I was still highly uncomfortable with my body—The weekly procedures and diagnostic testing were unbelievably awkward and embarrassing. . . . I followed [the doctors'] orders, but with the intention that I would soon return to normal. When [the symptoms] didn't leave, I added resentment to my feelings of invasion, awkwardness, and discomfort. . . . I force myself to rationalize the need for my continual doctor visits. . . . However, in all of my rationality, I cannot rid myself of the feeling of indignation and annoyance at physicians who are allowed to invade and control my body. Physicians must realize the sacredness of personal space and of independence and should be aware that some [patients] cherish those immensely.

A senior wrote about her back and abdominal pain, undiagnosed for years, despite multiple tests. Physicians did not believe her; they discounted her pain. Among the worst things that can happen to a patient, she learned, is a sense that physicians mistrust her observations about her own body. "My anger [with physicians about their inability to diagnose the cause of the pain] somewhere along the way was turned into energy. If no one could tell me the problem, I would have to learn as much as possible so one day I could diagnose myself. After all, I know the pain best."

A sophomore felt the impact of her younger brother's illness and death from a brain tumor on her (she was 9 at the time), her family, and the medical staff.

Even through countless spinal taps, surgeries, treatments with potent drugs, and days and nights in the hospital, [he] amazed everyone he came into contact with. He was cheerful and brave and sweet and optimistically drew pictures of himself beating up the bad cancer cells. . . . [After he died] I refused to talk about his death with anyone, and I never cried. I was enrolled in several counseling sessions, which I refused to attend. . . . The images I keep in my head have not faded in the ten years since his death. I remember seeing nurses cheerfully joke with him in his hospital room, and I watched as they went around the corner to cry. I saw doctors weep openly with my family as they talked about his prognosis. At age 9, these images taught me that adults, even nurses and doctors, were not immune to sorrow, and that they couldn't make everything better in the end after all.

In recalling her grandmother's illness, ovarian cancer, a senior discovered that each family member experienced the illness in different ways, that the drama of the illness became part of the larger drama of family life, and that it is important for families to care for the one who is ill, but equally important to take care of each other.

Perhaps her final gift to us was to unite and bind us all [together] like we hadn't ever been before. We learned how to take care of each other. I learned how to listen to someone, even when she can't speak. I think in today's society, we are raised with a focus on individualism, independence. That sense . . . is blown apart when you don't have any control over what is going on around you. I learned from this experience that in times of uncertainty, you need to lean on people, become dependent, and that that's okay to do.

Illness provokes fear, not limited to the patient. Recalling his childhood seizure disorder, a junior wrote:

My dad once told me that he had never been so scared in his life as he was when I started having my seizures. . . . I learned that people who suffer from illnesses, especially kids, are incredibly dependent on family members for support and assistance, and that those people who provide the assistance have their own fears and doubts regarding the illness. Sometimes, these even surpass the fears and doubts of the patient.

In telling the story of his grandfather's heart surgery, a senior understood that the physician ought to be more than a technician.

During the period of time leading up to the surgery, [my grandfather] frequently expressed frustration with his physician, who did not seem to spend much time with him or explain what was happening in easily understood terms. . . . After the surgery, [he] had the challenge of both recovering his strength as well as coming to terms with the fact [that] he would not be able to be as active as he was prior to the operation. . . . My grandfather's postoperative experience also served as a reinforcement to my long-held belief that although it is important to take care of the body, the mental state of a patient can have a profound effect on his or her physical condition and recovery as well. The mental aspect of patient care is easily and frequently lost in allopathic medicine.

Insights come from all kinds of illness, common and rare. Too often, we define a person by a single attribute. Physicians' goals are to learn all that they can about each patient. The teacher's task is to reinforce the desire and the ability to get the details of each patient's story. The following story teaches the importance of discovering more about the person because that information helps to plan treatment. Of her grandmother's obesity, a junior wrote:

Her condition is disabling and prevents her from any physical activity, with the exception of walking distances less than one block. Her lack of exercise has caused complications related to her obesity, such as diabetes and chronic digestive problems. . . . My grandmother's illness stems from psychological issues which were never addressed. She grew up during the depression with not enough to eat. She tells stories of being hit before being put to bed so that she would feel pain, not hunger. She tells of teachers who told her mother she was too thin and should eat more; her mother responded by saying she already ate like a horse and did not need more food. And still, fifty to sixty years later, these stories bring tears to my grandmother's eyes.

Quite obviously the causes of my grandmother's illness have not been properly addressed. Perhaps doctors have only advised remedies, such as diets she will never follow and exercise she will never do, without addressing the causes of her illness. Or perhaps my grandmother is too afraid to face her fear of not having enough to eat. Her fear is understandable when you consider that her generation was taught that psychological weakness or illness was shameful and should never be acknowledged.

A recurring theme in many of the students' stories is the intertwining of the physical and the psychological. A senior wrote of her experience with ulcerative colitis:

Over the following six years [after the diagnosis], I underwent a number of "relapses," which resulted in repeat hospitalizations, and another half-dozen major surgeries. Complication upon complication arose, from excessive scar tissue formation to postsurgical abscesses, and it seemed I would never lead a normal life. Somewhere in my midteens I began experiencing what I now recognize as clinical depression, likely resulting from my chronic ill health on top of a difficult home life. I strongly believe that the hardships I faced both emotionally and physically existed (and perpetuated one another) in a cyclical fashion. In an odd way, however, my struggle with ulcerative colitis changed my life in more positive ways than negative ones.

A sophomore's experience teaches us that even young people can handle the challenges of illness. Yet the concerns of chronic illness continue to preoccupy them and their families.

In terms of emotions, I would have to say that the best part of my experience with diabetes for both my family and for me has been my ability to take responsibility for my own health, even at an early age. I believe that my own initiative took much of the worry off of my parents onto me. However, my parents recently admitted to me that there has always been a corner in their minds that is devoted purely to worrying about my health and dreading the possibility of their daughter dying at an early age. This worry has been with me personally for many years, taking on more or less significance depending on my stage in life. In a nutshell, the best part of this experience has been hope; and the worst part has been fear.

Some students even had insights about how denial and guilt may be part of patients' stories. Of his experience with diabetes, a senior wrote: "Although these symptoms [blurred vision, thirst, frequent urination, weight loss] were clearly not normal, my mom seemed to refuse to believe something was wrong. . . . My mom at one point told me that I could have died from her negligence and that she felt very remorseful for not acting appropriately."

When her brother, a third grader, broke his leg in a sledding accident and required surgery, a junior learned that unless the medical system and the physician attend to the human side of medicine and keep an open mind, the patient and the family can suffer needlessly. One unsympathetic hospital staff person regarded her brother as "being a baby" for complaining about pain; the pain was real and was caused by an orthopedic pin that needed to be readjusted.

My mother . . . felt like she had to monitor everything that went on and keep asking questions and checking everything out. . . . [My brother's] time in the hospital has convinced me that someone who is seriously sick or in the hospital needs to have a person, a guardian so to speak, to ask questions. . . . The person who is sick may be incapable or too close to the situation to do it by himself.

Collectively, these students' stories supply sufficient content for a course about the human side of medicine. They are more dramatic than any tabulated information and valuable lessons for any doctor. The ease with which the students tell their stories in a trusting environment provides a model for a trusting relationship with a physician. The students' reflections validate their innate humanity and sensitivity and help to define part of the teacher's task in the training of physicians: to nourish and reinforce those qualities and do nothing to subtract from them.

These last chapters suggest many of the elements of what it is like to be a patient. In the next chapters, I will explore two of them in depth: uncertainty and how patients and their families deal with illness.

Chapter 6

Learning about Uncertainty

"Nobody is that precise. . . . The idea is to use your best stuff."

Patients and physicians alike would agree that one of the hardest parts of experiencing illness is the uncertainty.[1] Patients can bear pain of great magnitude—the pain of childbirth, for instance—when they know the cause and that the outcome will be good, but lesser pains may be overwhelming when there are unanswered questions about the diagnosis, the treatment, or the prognosis. Many physicians struggle not so much with a patient's illness going badly but rather with their own questions of uncertainty: Have I overlooked a possible diagnosis? Have I chosen the best treatment? What information am I lacking?

Seasoned physicians understand that uncertainty is a part of most encounters with illness, but for those new to the experience—a patient or a family never before faced with a serious illness or a physician just beginning—the uncertainties are magnified. Yet we act even in the face of uncertainty. Uncertainty need not paralyze action.

A PATIENT'S HISTORY AND THE UNCERTAINTIES

This brief medical history seems straightforward:

A 66-year-old man told his physician that he was having chest pain. After cancer of the esophagus was diagnosed, he had surgery, radiation, and chemotherapy. Two years later, he was feeling well, with no recurrence of his tumor.

Yet this history is filled with uncertainties. Here are the details.

A 66-year-old man told his physician that he had been having intermittent mild chest pains for three months, occurring both at rest and with activity. When his cardiac stress test was normal, his physician investigated other possible causes for the pain. Gastrointestinal x-rays and endoscopy [examining the esophagus, stomach, and duodenum with a special instrument] confirmed the presence of esophageal cancer.

At the beginning, the patient wonders, "Is this pain, not very severe, worth seeing a physician about?" After the diagnosis is made, he wonders, "How will this turn out? Am I going to die? If I survive, will I be the same person? How will my family manage? Where should I have the surgery—in my hometown hospital or at the medical center?"

The physician's uncertainties begin with diagnosis. He asks, "Where's the disease? Is this the pain of unstable angina, which requires urgent investigation, or can the evaluation be delayed for a few days to see what happens?" When the cardiac stress test shows that the pain is not caused by coronary artery disease, he wonders, "Should I look for other causes? Where else could the disease be? In the esophagus? In the gallbladder? Could stress cause the pain?"

The patient underwent complex and extensive surgery: resection of much of the esophagus, removal of the tumor through both a chest and an abdominal incision, and placement of part of his stomach within the chest cavity to establish a connection between the remaining esophagus and the stomach. Two days following surgery, he became very apprehensive. The nurse discovered that his blood pressure was low and called his physician.

The uncertainties for the nurse: What is the cause of his apprehension? Is he simply anxious, or are there other reasons including low blood pressure and infection?

The uncertainties for the physician: Is the blood pressure drop due to hemorrhage, to dehydration, or to a myocardial infarct (heart attack)? What are the priorities in resolving the dilemma? What should I do first?

An electrocardiogram was normal and showed no evidence of a myocardial infarct. Hemoglobin determination suggested dehydration rather than hemorrhage. When the blood pressure returned to normal after additional intravenous fluids were administered, the patient's apprehension resolved. The next day, the report of the microscopic study of the tumor showed cancer cells at the edge of the resection.

The uncertainties for the physician: To what extent do these microscopic findings influence the prognosis? What are the treatment options? Will they help or make the patient feel worse? Of all the options, radiation and/or chemotherapy or no additional treatment at all, which should I recommend if I am uncertain of the outcome of treatment? How completely should I share these uncertainties with the patient and his wife?

The uncertainties for the patient: If there are no guarantees about the success of additional treatment and I might feel worse yet from it, should I take a chance on squandering time on useless therapy? Should I get another opinion? His wife shares all of these concerns.

The patient, his wife, and his physician spoke frankly about the uncertainties and agreed on additional treatment, which included radiation and chemotherapy. Three months later, after completing treatment, he noticed difficulty swallowing, which lasted for several days.

The uncertainties for the patient: What does this swallowing difficulty mean? Is my tumor back? Have all of this surgery and additional treatment been for nothing? The physician faces the same questions, but also asks, "Other than recurrent cancer, what else could be causing the difficulty? Could it be from a scarred narrowing of the esophagus from the surgery or irradiation, from an ulcer or an inflamed esophagus?"

Once again, the patient had endoscopy, which showed a narrowed scar at the site of the connection between the esophagus and stomach. After the endoscopist dilated the stricture, the symptom resolved. A month later, the patient developed chest pain, which lasted for a day. He called his physician, who felt that the pain was of no consequence. He acknowledged the patient's concerns and told him, "Sometimes, the best test is the test of time. Likely this is not serious. Let's wait a few days and see what happens." The pain resolved.

His physician saw him periodically thereafter, not only to review his interval story and examine him but also to address his uncertainties and provide support and perspective. Two years later, the patient was feeling well. The patient, his wife, and his physician understand that his disease, cancer of the esophagus, may not be cured and requires ongoing surveillance.

WHAT DO WE LEARN?

What do we learn from this patient's story? What are the issues that relate to uncertainty? What are the opportunities to enhance his care? What lessons do we learn from this story that help us care for other patients? All who are involved with the drama of the patient's illness—in this case, the patient, his wife, his physicians and nurses—may be dealing with different dimensions of uncertainty.

For patients, uncertainty is part of most illnesses and symptoms. The uncertainty may be related to diagnosis, treatment, prognosis, or all of these. A patient with swollen lymph nodes may worry that she has cancer. A patient with a fractured ankle may be concerned that his pain after surgery means that he has an infection or that the fracture is displaced again. And so, *no matter how trivial the illness or symptom, physicians should make some statement regarding diagnosis, proposed treatment, and prognosis.* Even when no serious illness is present, physicians can conclude the transaction by saying, "I think that this will turn out all right" or "I think this pain will resolve in a few days."

Physicians can authorize patients to acknowledge their uncertainties. They can say, "You wouldn't be human if you were not apprehensive about your upcoming surgery." They can ask, "What concerns you the most about this illness? Having been ill for so long, you must have had your own thoughts about what's wrong. What are they?" By encouraging patients to express themselves, doctors can discover unrecognized fears and needs.

Being unjustifiably certain can cause harm. Had the physician prematurely concluded that the first episodes of chest pain were angina and not arranged for the other tests, he would have squandered precious time and the opportunity for effective treatment of the esophageal cancer.

Recognizing uncertainty stimulates creative thought. If this patient's chest pain was not angina, what else could it be? If the posttreatment swallowing difficulty was not caused by recurrent cancer, what other treatable condition could it be?

Physicians especially need to attend to apprehension and anxiety in the midst of illness. Although this patient's apprehension was caused by dehydration and low blood pressure, anxiety may represent a patient's unspoken struggle with uncertainty about diagnosis, treatment, and outcome. Physicians often regard such patients as "difficult patients," when they really should be asking, "Do we create difficult patients because we don't talk frankly about uncertainty?"

Physicians' uncertainties may be multidimensional. Experienced physicians may not know initially the diagnosis, the best treatment, or the prognosis. Physicians-in-training often feel uncertain because of inexperience. Unable to answer a question, they may not recognize the difference between not knowing because of lack of knowledge or because there simply is no answer; that is, the critical discovery has yet to be made. But physicians have many resources, and the ethic of medicine authorizes, encourages, and obligates them to consult with colleagues when uncertain and to provide advice when asked. One need not be reluctant to ask for advice. Medicine is a collaborative profession.

Physicians can share their uncertainty with the patient without undermining the trusting relationship. The greater the trust, the easier it is for the patient to handle uncertainty. Uncertainty is a reality of everyday life, and most patients are sufficiently wise to recognize the parallels related to health and illness. Patients can accept uncertainty when their doctors understand their needs, respect their intelligence, and explain carefully. This patient trusted his physician when he suggested the "test of time" for his later episode of chest pain. Here are some other ways to speak with patients about uncertainty:

- For a patient with abdominal pain: "While I'm not certain what's causing your pain, I don't believe this is anything of a serious nature. Call me in a few days if it's not better, sooner if it gets worse. Are you comfortable with that approach?"

- For a patient who is faced with choosing a treatment from a number of difficult choices: "Each choice has some benefits and some risks. This is what I think is the best choice. How do you feel about it?"

We can make choices and take action in the face of uncertainty. In this drama, the patient, his wife, and his physician struggled through the dilemmas together. In this shared undertaking, each identified and acknowledged the uncertainties to the others, made decisions, and took action. Even though there were no guarantees of a good outcome, they made choices. They all recognized that no choice was irrevocable and that decisions could be altered as the drama evolved.

Put another way, *if we strive for certainty before we take action, we may become paralyzed.* In practice, a physician faces many points of decision each day. Some require immediate action, but each alternative, if a wrong one, may delay recovery or jeopardize the patient's well-being. Physicians solve the dilemma by making the best decision they can, trying it out, making observations to test the validity of the decision, and, if need be, altering the decision.

The Minnesota Twins ace pitcher from the 1970s, Dave Goltz, once said, "A pitcher can try to be too fine, or some other people can expect him to be too fine. But nobody is that precise with every pitch. The idea is to use your best stuff and be confident it will work out."[2] Scientist-philosopher Jacob Bronowski saw that "errors are inextricably bound up with the nature of human knowledge."[3] To that I add, errors are inextricably bound up with the nature of human behavior and judgments.

Even when there are no technical matters to deal with, no treatment to alter, and no tests to monitor, periodic encounters help to identify and address the patient's concerns and uncertainties, and that is an important part of patient care. Patients struggle to address their questions and uncertainties, often long after they have gone beyond their ability to do so. Physicians can encourage patients to share their struggle by telling them, "If you can't figure out what to do about your pain [or your blood sugar, etc.], call me." Doctors can acknowledge to patients that "the hardest part of your illness, I know, is the uncertainty. Let me know when you need help."

TEACHING ABOUT UNCERTAINTY

I give students this written assignment:

1. Look to your own experience and describe an event in your own life where uncertainty was or is a substantial element. What were the choices? What were the issues? Could you take action despite *not* knowing for sure all the facts and not having all the data? How did you handle it? What was it like for you? What did you do to deal with the dilemma? What was the outcome?
2. Discuss in a similar way a medical situation from your own experience or that of someone in your family where uncertainty was a prominent element.
3. What do you learn as you reflect on your answers?

In addressing these questions, students have described a variety of situations: choosing a college, choosing a career, moving from one country to another, or dealing with an unplanned pregnancy, a sibling with a brain tumor, a mother's depression, or parents' divorce. They have learned about "the strength of human character in the face of uncertainty," that "uncertainty . . . is just a part of life . . . [and that] an appropriate level of uncertainty can actually enhance an experience," that "in medicine, as in all other aspects of life, no one can be 100 percent sure of any diagnosis, efficacy of treatment, or prognosis. Every situation is different, and so we can only make our best educated guesses at what choices are wise and how they will ultimately unfold." Students have recognized that the uncertainty is an almost universal presence in medical matters.

Dealing with uncertainty is an important part of physicians' work. Despite uncertainty regarding diagnosis, treatment, and prognosis, physicians take action. Experience teaches them how to share the uncertainty of illness with patients and families in ways that do not undermine trust and confidence. To strive for certainty and perfection is an admirable and uniquely human task. We need not abandon that goal so long as we recognize that imperfection and uncertainty are equally human. The next chapter deals with the variety of ways in which patients handle the uncertainty, stress, and losses of illness.

Chapter 7

Learning How Patients Handle Illness

"I needed to be in control of my disease."

Perceptive physicians continually find themselves awestruck by how patients and their families cope with illness and injury. Those doctors who do not take the time to listen and learn from their stories squander the opportunity to grow professionally and provide crucial support.

How do patients handle bad news? Does the physician have to be reluctant to deliver bad news? What can we learn from examining these questions? For a class session, I invite speakers from CanSurmount, a group of volunteers who have had cancer treatment and now counsel patients with newly diagnosed malignancy similar to their own. My request of them is a simple one: "During this session, I hope that we can help the students see the diversity of ways that patients handle serious illness. What do you ask of your physician and of others who are involved in your care?" Each of the speakers has had a variety of tests and treatments, including surgery, chemotherapy, radiation, and bone marrow transplantation. Each mode of therapy has been rigorous, with unpleasant side effects. The speakers describe their experience: what it was like, what some of their losses were, and their relationship with their physicians. Here are excerpts from their stories.

One man was 41 years old when lymphoma was diagnosed, and he had chemotherapy and a bone marrow transplant.

With cancer, you can feel good one day, bad the next . . . The first doctor said, "It's cancer; it's not serious; you'll need two doses of chemotherapy." The second doctor said, "It's stage IV [the most serious stage], treatable, not curable, non-Hodgkin's lymphoma." He went on [with what he was saying], but I was on page 1 while he was on page 5. . . . I don't know if compassion can be taught. When they're dealing with cancer, doctors need to slow down, to take the time with people, to talk the same language, to ask if [the patients] understand. . . . Everybody else thought I was doing great, but no one knew how I really felt. . . . I was really scared for my family. . . . The biggest thing is the uncertainty, what is going to happen to my family and me. . . . There are things that have happened to me that have been harder than cancer.

A 25-year-old woman was told she had cancer of the ovary when she was 23. After her second operation, she developed pneumonia and peritonitis, a serious abdominal infection.

[It's] not just that I had cancer . . . but so much more. . . . I can't have kids. . . . I had memory loss from chemotherapy. . . . What do I ask of my physician? Be positive. Give me hope. One doctor said, "There's a 50–50 chance and that's all I'd give you." [My response was]: "If you're going to focus on statistics, and not on me, I'll change doctors." Be honest. Tell me everything. Tell me over and over again. Tell me about side effects. If I know it's a possibility, I can deal with it later on. Tell me about support groups. Encourage people to go into support groups. If I ask for a second opinion, I'd rather not have my physician threatened by that. Give me a good joke. . . . My dad blamed himself because [the cancer history] was [on] his side of the family.

A middle-aged woman spoke about her illness, non-Hodgkin's lymphoma, which had been diagnosed twenty-four years previously.

It was a great shock to look at marriage, birth, and death all at once, in a very short time. . . . [I found] something to live for in our daughter. . . . My physician and I were a good match. She knew it and I knew it. . . . A lot of physical changes took place in my body [as a result of the treatment]: instant menopause, no more children. . . . What I wanted to know right away was a lot of information. I was looking for causes. Why? What can I do to prevent it [from recurring]? . . . There were many wonderful people: the physician, a good family support system. It was hard for my mother. . . . I had a strong faith background. The pastor asked, "Do you want people to know?" Back then there was a stigma [about having cancer]. . . . My physician wanted to know about me as a person. [She told me], "This is treatable." . . . She was very honest. [She told me] the truth, with hope. . . . When you have cancer, you feel like a lot of things are out of your control, so when there is the opportunity for choice, you want it. . . . I don't believe I realized what it was like for my husband. . . . He saw his role as looking after our child . . . protecting me . . . limiting me from wallowing. . . . [In dealing with other problems in our lives], we can look back on our experience [with my cancer] and say, "We went through this together."

He was 28 when he was given the diagnosis, non-Hodgkin's lymphoma, after he noticed some abnormal lumps. He had been nauseated for about six months, but he thought the cause of the nausea was the nearby sewage treatment plant.

[The doctor said], "Looks like you got yourself cancer." I didn't want the medical jargon. I needed things in layman's terms, an optimistic approach, what to look forward to with side effects. . . . Doctors became a support group. . . . Humor was important. . . . On day 1 I asked, "Why did this happen to me? . . . Life goes downhill very fast. . . . The doctor said, "This is a common cancer. Your prognosis is very good." . . . I wondered, "Am I still going to have a job?" . . . Everybody—friends, co-workers, religion, doctors, people I'd never met—becomes your support group. Others don't want to be with you. . . . Chemotherapy was very intimidating at first. I had no idea what it was. . . . I had loss of energy, loss of hair, not as bad for guys. . . . I didn't want my family to have to see me die. . . . I planned my death. I put photo albums together. I wrote my obituary.

When stage IV non-Hodgkin's lymphoma was diagnosed, she was 33. Her symptoms were lumps, fatigue, and night sweats.

I knew I was sick but I had trouble getting someone to believe me. . . . The hot flashes and tiredness . . . were all explained away because I was a woman. . . . [After the biopsy], I called the clinic, because no one had called me. [When the doctor spoke to me], I think he was reading the report for the first time. . . . I had nine months of chemotherapy. I threw up a lot, but I felt better a lot. . . . When I was retested, the chemotherapy had helped, but it still hadn't been complete. . . . I had a bone marrow transplant. [The initial encounter with the physician at the medical center was] the worst encounter I ever had. The doctor just rattled off statistics like I wasn't a person, just a statistic. . . . [After the bone marrow transplant] when they told me there was a "2 percent gray area," it wasn't fair that they couldn't tell me I was 100 percent cured. . . . I was depressed and I saw a psychiatrist and a psychologist. [Later I was told], "not a trace of cancer." . . . Now I live for [each] day. . . . It's two years in remission. . . . I'm very cautious about my future.

Before her diagnosis of ovarian cancer, when she first started to feel ill, "the doctor thought I had some kind of infection." When her symptoms persisted, she went to a hospital emergency room.

[I knew] I needed some help. . . . [After examining me and doing some tests], the emergency room doctor told me, "You have a bowel obstruction, but that's not the real cause. You have cancer." . . . The three days between admission and surgery were valuable days, meetings with the oncologist and the surgeon, the opportunity to educate myself. . . . It was important to have some time to think about it . . . to speak to my parents, to put my business on hold, for my husband to read about [my diagnosis]. . . . The nurses gave me huge amounts of information regarding chemotherapy. . . . I needed to have a lot of information. . . . I needed to be in control of my disease. The doctor xeroxed everything. It was important for me to read this, to see their evaluation, to read it at my leisure. . . . I liked the second oncologist better. He believed very much in treating me as a whole person. [He told me], "I need to know how you're feeling. Call me anytime." He recognized how much control I needed. . . . I was waiting to hear the word "curable." . . . I read in the doctor's notes, "The patient understands that the disease is incurable." . . . I know that I have the disease that will ultimately kill me. . . . My husband and I coped in various ways. As we waited for the results of the tests, we asked ourselves, "What is the worst that can happen, the best that can happen?" You can cope with something in between. . . . We did not think too far ahead. . . . We avoided asking, "What if?" . . . We deal with it in chunks of time. I would encourage physicians not to deal with too much at a time. . . . I felt cheated that it had happened to me so young.

WHAT DO WE LEARN?

Physicians' contacts with patients occur in short encounters, often lasting no more than fifteen minutes. But their story evolves during the intervals between doctor visits, and we may know nothing about the larger drama unless we ask. Physicians can enhance their patients' ability to cope with the burdens of illness by appreciating how they handle illness and what they need from physicians. Here are some lessons from the patients' stories.

Patients need to be seen as individuals and not narrowly defined as "cancer patients." They need compassion and repeated expressions of understanding and empathy. They need a consistent message, not conflicting information from different physicians. They need a clear, jargon-free explanation about what to expect from their illness and the treatment, but not so much information all at once that they are overwhelmed. Important information needs to be repeated. They need hope, even in the face of uncertainty. Sometimes they need humor.

Patients need time. They may be devastated by the diagnosis, but then they mobilize their strengths and resources. During the interval between being informed of a diagnosis and beginning treatment, patients think, study, and talk things over with others. They begin to accept change brought about by the illness and learn how to cope with the change. They integrate the experience of their illness into the longer story of their life, and they review the story of their own lives and ways in which they have coped with other crises.

Patients need a sense of control, not so much to "be in charge" as a feeling that their situation is not "out of control." When there are choices to be made, they want a role in making them. Even though the physician has the technical expertise, most patients need to be partners in making the important decisions.

Serious illness often represents many losses—loss of energy, loss of control, loss of independence—and the disruption of the rhythm of one's life and day-to-day activities. There may be loss of contact with others; illness can be very isolating. Relationships are disrupted; serious illness can precipitate divorce. In response to illness, well-meaning family and friends often do not know what to do, how to behave, how to inquire, and how to provide support. There is loss of status; even well-meaning people can be patronizing.

It does not necessarily follow that because people have cancer, they will become depressed. If depression is present, the physician should address that as a separate problem. Most people are able to talk about their illness and their feelings, but some cannot. If they cannot, then the role of the physician is to help patients express themselves. It is better than guessing.

Patients cope in different ways. The role of the family is important. Over and over, we learn that illness is a family affair. Some patients can rely on family and some cannot. Some can rely on their physicians; others cannot. There are other sources of support: faith, religion, and philosophy of life; a strong inner self—what one student described as "inner serenity"; the workplace with its people and its routines; friends; favored activities and hobbies; pets; literature; and psychotherapy. Individuals who have had a similar illness can help. They especially know the details of the illness, the ups and the downs, the nuances of physical and emotional feelings, what can go wrong, and what minor symptoms mean. Support groups can help.

Even if one is not "religious," most patients have a spiritual dimension to their lives, which provides yet another resource for dealing with illness. They see and seek meaning and metaphor in their illness, sometimes without even knowing it. They express it in different ways; they say "I'm being punished" or "It isn't fair." Every illness is a potential spiritual crisis; finding meaning in illness is a worthwhile pursuit. Denying patients the opportunity to address the spiritual dimensions of illness is a disservice to them. Searching for meaning in illness is potentially enriching for patients and for professionals.

A physician can discover how patients cope and what their strengths are by listening carefully to their stories. If there are specific questions to ask to encourage patients to talk, these are the obvious ones: "What's this like for you? How's your morale? How have you dealt with crisis in the past? Who do you turn to for moral support? Who is your community? Where do you find your strength?"

But not all patients and their families cope well and find relief. Not all resolve their fears and uncertainties and address their feelings. Those situations provide physicians and others yet another opportunity to intervene in a way that is healing, enriching, and strengthening for the patient and the family. While much of the time, the patient is the center of the drama, sometimes other important dramas are going on in the patient's family, and complex relationships need to be explored. Do we know the whole story? Do we really understand what it is like?

Only when we focus on the patient's experience do we begin to appreciate the richness, depth, and challenge of being a physician. The next section deals with what it is like to be a physician and begins with the diary of one day in the life of a doctor.

PART II

WHAT IT'S LIKE TO BE A PHYSICIAN

Chapter 8

A Day in the Life of a Physician

"What do doctors do all day?"

When they were small, my kids liked reading a book with this question in the title: "What do people do all day?"[1] I ask now, "What do doctors do all day?" Copies of my hospital and office chart notes from 1992 provide this diary of one of my days. The hospital notes were handwritten; the office notes were dictated after each transaction, while the information was fresh in my mind. Dictating, rather than writing longhand, was a great time saver and enabled me to describe the patients' problems, the data, and my reflections in more detail.

Each note begins with the "history" of the illness, and each part of the history is titled with the name of the problem. The name focuses the note and my thinking as I integrate the data and make decisions. In this chapter, many of the notes will be followed by a brief commentary, sampling and explaining the italicized medical terms and jargon, some of the shorthand of medicine. These comments also take advantage of the "teachable moment," when there is a need for explanation and an opportunity to learn. To preserve privacy, I have altered some of the details about patients and given them fictitious initials. The notes are in the order in which I dealt with them, and the reader can refer back and forth between this chapter and chapter 22, where I provide a different type of commentary, one that examines in greater detail part of the patient's story and additional history, the derivative issues, and the role of the doctor-patient relationship and then addresses the question, "What did I learn?"

Read the chart notes with the recognition that no day is typical and that physicians' practices differ according to their specialty, their specific interests, and how they choose to practice. The universal quality of all practices is the diversity of patients and problems physicians see in any day.

I began my day at the hospital at 7:30 a.m., took thirty minutes for lunch at 12:30 p.m., and was home for dinner by 6 p.m. The evening's house call took an hour.

THE HOSPITAL

Patient 1: A.B., Age 29

Abdominal pain and weight loss: Still no appetite. Tests, including proctoscopy, barium enema, endoscopy of stomach, and CT scan of abdomen, show a small ovarian mass. Thyroid tests are normal.

Seizures: now and then.

Her abdominal pain and weight loss are very likely multidetermined—related to her antiseizure medication and the psychosocial issues in her life. Prior to discharge, we need to settle the medication issue and arrange for adequate psychiatric follow-up.

Patient 2: C.D., Age 85

Back pain: persists. X-ray shows *osteoporosis* of the lumbar spine and old compression fractures but no new ones. Her exam is unchanged. *She rarely requires pain medication.*

Commentary: *Osteoporosis:* Abnormally fragile bones. *She . . . medication:* That is, she is improving.

Patient 3: E.F., Age 85

Fever and lightheadedness: She's no longer lightheaded. Fever has disappeared. Potassium deficit: has been corrected.

Patient 4: G.H., Age 78

Fever: improving. No cough, no chills. Urinalysis is normal. Chest x-ray normal.

Diabetes mellitus: Blood sugars are in the 100–200 range on a mixture of *NPH and regular insulin*.

Coronary heart disease: no breathlessness, no chest pain, no significant arrhythmia.

Thought disorder: He is still combative, and he won't talk to me.

Exam: Alert, *does not look acutely ill*. Chest: clear. Heart: regular rhythm.

Etiology of the fever is still unclear, though he is improving on intravenous antibiotic.

Commentary: *NPH and regular insulin*: Two different varieties of insulin, each with a different duration of action. "100–200" ranges from normal to an elevated level of blood sugar concentration. *Thought disorder*: A specific broad category of mental illness. Mental illness is an important portion of what physicians see in their daily practice. Some require consultation from a psychiatrist or other mental health professional. *does . . . ill*: Despite his multitude of problems, he does not *look* sick, and that is important information, as any mother can tell you. I learned that this is an important observation to make from one of my pediatric instructors in medical school; it will appear in many of the notes.

Patient 5: I.J., Age 68

Congestive heart failure: Overall he feels much better. Not breathless. Slept well. He has lost 10 pounds since admission, on varying doses of *furosemide*.

Exam: Pulse 60, irregular. Blood pressure 120/80. He weeps as he speaks of his illnesses. *Neck veins flat at 30 degrees*. Chest: clear. Heart: irregular rhythm, variable *S-1* as before. Liver: not palpable. No presacral or pretibial edema.

Gout: *Erythema* and pain in his hand have resolved.

Pelvic tumor: no symptoms.

Commentary: *Furosemide*: A diuretic medicine, one that increases the urinary output of excessive body fluid. I will, for the most part, use uncapitalized names for generic drugs and capitalize brandnames. *Neck . . . 30 degrees*: The extent of jugular vein distension, when the patient lies with trunk elevated 30 degrees from a flat surface. Here the finding indicates improvement in his congestive heart failure. *S-1*: The first of two sounds of the heartbeat. *Erythema*: The appearance of redness, often a sign of infection or inflammation.

THE OFFICE

From the hospital, I went to my office, where my day is a mixture of transactions:

- "Complete physicals," a review with patients of their entire medical history, followed by a physical examination from top to toe, discussion of all the material with the patients, and planning any necessary follow-up. Each such encounter lasts from forty-five minutes to an hour.

- Shorter visits with established patients, averaging about fifteen minutes.

- Telephone calls interspersed between patient visits. These calls may come from patients, nurses caring for patients in the hospital or in nursing homes, and occasionally family members.

- Talking things over with the staff—a receptionist, a laboratory technician, a transcriber—and my partner, another internist.

Patient 6: K.L., Age 45

A 45-year-old woman here for annual physical. Problems are as follows:

Myxomatous mitral valve, post mitral valve replacement: on *warfarin*. No chest pain. No breathlessness. No awareness of irregular heartbeat. *EKG* today shows *sinus bradycardia*, rate about 56, with frequent *ventricular extrasystoles* and *first degree a-v block*.

Thought disorder: ongoing.

Weight loss: a new problem. Weight 14 months ago was 150 and now is 138. She says she is struggling financially and often does not eat well. No special weather preference to suggest *hyperthyroidism*.

Medications: warfarin and some over-the-counter health-food preparations.

Review of systems is otherwise essentially negative.

Psychosocial: Though she is struggling financially, she does not consistently turn to anyone for moral support. She knows that she can rely on her niece.

(In this and the one subsequent "complete physical," I have eliminated the description of the physical exam, which is quite detailed. In the subsequent notes, the physical examination is focused on the pertinent issues, is briefer, and is included.)

Impression: Weight loss, probably due to inadequate nutrition. Urged to eat better.

Arrhythmia, as noted above. Probably not *clinically significant*.

With her permission, I will speak with her niece.

Return in 3 months.

Commentary: *Myxomatous mitral valve*: Abnormal tissue in the heart's mitral valve, sometimes causing poor valve function and predisposing to congestive heart failure. *warfarin*: A drug that reduces the clotting ability of the blood and the risk of blood clots. EKG: Electrocardiogram. *sinus bradycardia*: A slow heart rate. *ventricular extrasystoles*: Irregular heartbeats that may or may not cause difficulty. *first-degree a-v block*: Atrial-ventricular block, a lengthening of the time required for contraction of the heart.

Sometimes this finding requires an alteration in therapy. *hyperthyroidism:* An overactive thyroid gland, one cause of weight loss. An intolerance to heat or a preference for cooler weather is a symptom that sometimes indicates hyperthyroidism. *Review of systems:* A litany of specific questions the physician asks the patient regarding symptoms related to each organ system of the body. *Impression:* This is the summary of my conclusions and includes statements of problems, which may be diagnoses or other kinds of problem statements such as yet-to-be-explained symptoms, findings on physical examination, or abnormal laboratory tests. *clinically significant:* Among the important judgments a physician makes is whether or not the abnormality significantly affects the patient's well-being or prognosis.

Patient 7: M.N., Age 50

A 50-year-old woman here for annual physical. Problems are as follows:

Diabetes mellitus: *no weakness, numbness, or tingling of face, arms or legs, nausea, diarrhea, change in vision.* She has periodic eye checkups by ophthalmologist and *retinologist.* No symptoms to suggest hypoglycemia. She is on this insulin regimen: regular insulin 12 to 18 units before breakfast, lunch, and supper, and NPH 30 units before supper. She does not regularly test her blood but chooses the amount of insulin according to how active she is going to be. She has given up sweets and finds that there are fewer swings in her blood sugar when she does test.

Hypertension: No headaches or dizziness. On Vasotec, 5 mg. daily.

Asthma: rare wheezing. She takes albuterol, 2 puffs, before she runs and as needed, and Theodur, 600 mg twice a day.

Caffeine excess: drinks about two cups of coffee a day and one or two cans of caffeinated cola a day.

Possible allergy to penicillin

Ethanol, nicotine, and drug excess: none for many years.

Rectal bleeding: none.

Epigastric burning: none.

Impaired hearing: unchanged.

Review of systems is otherwise essentially negative.

Psychosocial: All in all, things are going well for her. She has taken on new work responsibilities, shares her feelings with her husband. She was offered a job in another city, actually the equivalent of a promotion, but chose to remain here.

Impression: Diabetes mellitus: adequate control for her. Check *Hgb A1C.*

Hypertension: adequately controlled.

Asthma: adequately controlled.

Plan: Continue current regimen. Call me in 4 days for test results and further discussion.

Commentary: *no weakness . . . vision:* In medical parlance, these are called "pertinent negatives," and in this case they relate to questions the physician specifically asks to determine whether the patient has any of the complications of diabetes. *retinologist:* An ophthalmologist who has special expertise in diseases of the retina. *Ethanol . . . years:* She had a previous active addiction. *Rectal . . . none; Epigastric . . . none:* She had previous symptoms that had been evaluated. The current appointment is an opportunity to review the interim progress of the symptoms. *Hgb A1C:* A blood test that is an index of how close to normal her blood sugar levels are and therefore one measure of adequate treatment for diabetes.

Patient 8: I.J., Age 68 (Telephone—Son)

We talked about some of the issues involved in his father's hospitalization (congestive heart failure, underlying heart disease, unusual tumor) and some of the uncertainties related to the illness.

Patient 9: O.P., Age 72 (Telephone)

Goiter: Repeat *TSH* is low. I spoke with my colleague, Dr. S and also with Dr. M, the radiation therapist, about further evaluation and treatment. The nodule is *"cold"* on the 1989 radioactive scan, but *thyroid aspiration* was normal. To repeat the scan now to look for any changes. Further decisions about treatment will be made after the scan.

Commentary: *TSH:* Thyroid-stimulating hormone, a blood test for thyroid function and often a measure of adequacy of thyroid hormone replacement treatment. *cold:* That is, metabolically inert, not producing thyroid hormone. Cold nodules are sometimes malignant. *thyroid aspiration:* Obtaining a sample of cells through a very thin needle to analyze them and look especially for signs of malignancy.

Patient 10: Q.R., Age 78 (Telephone)

Tongue biopsy was negative for malignancy, she says. Call as needed.

Patient 11: S.T., Age 46

Abnormal liver tests: *Gamma GT* done 3 days ago was 67. The trend is certainly not getting worse and is better than last time.

Exam: BP 130/80. Does not look ill. Chest: clear. Heart: regular rhythm. Abdomen: soft. Liver: not palpable.

The liver test abnormality is probably of no clinical significance. No further follow-up seems warranted. Recheck in a year.

Wart: She has a wart on her finger for which she is using Compound W and has some dry skin on her fingers for which she may use skin moistener.

Commentary: *Gamma GT:* A liver test. *Wart:* Not all problems for which patients seek physicians' advice are complex.

Patient 12: U.V., Age 58 (Telephone)

Elevated cholesterol: I spoke with her about her elevated cholesterol and will send her a diet. Recheck *lipid profile* in 3 months.

Nodules: She had the nodules excised and they were benign.

Commentary: *Lipid profile:* Test to measure blood levels of cholesterol and triglycerides (lipids). Lipids are fats.

Patient 13: W.X., Age 58 (Telephone)

We reviewed the instructions of yesterday. May stop Lactinex if stools firm up.

Commentary: *We . . . yesterday:* He has a complex illness. Sometimes instructions have to be repeated or clarified.

Patient 14: Y.Z., Age 72

Polymyalgia rheumatica: Muscle and joint aching persist. He feels as bad as when he entered the hospital in December. On prednisone 8 mg a day.

Exam: BP 140/80, P 80. Does not look acutely ill. He is *cushingoid*.

Hemoglobin: 13.6. *Sedimentation rate:* 43. *Electrolytes:* renal function tests OK.

Increase prednisone to 10 mg daily. Prescription for 5-mg tabs, #60, 2 each a.m. Call in 6 days.

Commentary: *Polymyalgia rheumatica:* A sometimes disabling illness characterized by muscle aching. *cushingoid:* He has the general appearance of someone who has Cushing's disease, caused by overproduction of cortisone, a hormone produced by the adrenal gland. One sees this appearance in a patient who has been taking prednisone, an artificial hormone similar to cortisone. *Sedimentation rate:* A blood test helpful in following the activity of polymyalgia rheumatica. *Electrolytes:* Blood test determination of the concentration of sodium, potassium, bicarbonate, and chloride, often done to look for adverse effects of medication. #60: That is, 60 tablets of predni-sone 5 mg. When I write a prescription, I record the number of pills pre-scribed. That helps me to evaluate whether the patient has been using the drug as directed or too frequently or infrequently. While such information is especially useful for drugs that are tranquilizers or narcotics, the informa-tion may be helpful with all drugs.

Patient 15: A.C., age 82 (Telephone–Nurse)

Blood sugars in the 200+ range on Micronase, 2.5 mg daily. Serum electrolytes: normal. BUN: 24 (was 17 in September). Creatinine: 1.2 (was 0.9 in September).

Take Micronase, 2.5 mg later today, then beginning tomorrow 5 mg daily. Call in 3 days with progress.

I spoke with her daughter to review her progress.

Commentary: BUN, Creatinine: Blood tests of kidney function. was . . . September: Often the comparison between values is as important as the ab-solute number.

Patient 16: B.D., Age 62 (Telephone)

Fatigue waxes and wanes. Continue current regimen. Call in 6 days.

Two issues need to be dealt with: (1) whether he needs further evaluation of his artificial aortic heart valve, and (2) whether he needs alteration in any medications that may be causing his fatigue.

Commentary: aortic heart valve: Which may have become damaged in the years since it was inserted.

Patient 17: C.E., Age 58

Hypertension: No headaches or dizziness. Premarin dose has been cut back to .625 mg daily 3 days ago.

Exam: BP 140/80. Does not look ill. Continue current regimen. Return 2 months.

Commentary: Premarin . . . ago: Because premarin, an artificial hormone, may cause hypertension, the physician previously advised the patient to re-duce the dose.

Patient 18: D.F., Age 88 (Telephone–Nurse)

All in all, doing well after hernia surgery. Bladder catheter has been removed, and he is voiding adequately.

Patient 19: E.G., Age 57 (Telephone)

Thyroid status: TSH 91+ 3 days ago. Increase Synthroid to 0.1 mg daily. Office in a month.

Commentary: TSH 91+: elevated, indicating need for more thyroid hormone.

Patient 20: F.H., Age 67 (Telephone)

He has a cough, which is evolving into symptoms of upper respiratory infection. Observe. Call if no better.

Patient 21: G.I., Age 78

Abdominal pain, colitis: She is feeling much better. She is having three bowel movements a day and she says they are more formed than before. She will shortly stop vancomycin.

Exam: BP 130/80, P 92. Does not look acutely ill. Chest: clear. Heart: regular rhythm. Abdomen: soft, nontender. Normal bowel sounds.

Continue azulfidine. She is to call in a week with progress. If no better, may con-sider specific antisalmonella treatment.

Patient 22: H.J., Age 74

Hypertension: no headaches. No dizziness. On Vasotec, 2.5 mg daily.

Exam: BP 140/80. Does not look ill. Continue Vasotec, 2.5 mg daily.

Abnormal prostate: He is anticipating prostate biopsy in a week and has a number of questions about the implications should malignancy be found and about the approach of his urologist. We discussed all of these issues at length.

Constipation: in the last month. Likely of no clinical consequence. He had colonoscopy 3 months ago. Prune juice seems to help.

Return 3 months.

Patient 23: I.K., Age 82 (Telephone–Nurse)

Toe ulcer: some *purulent* drainage. Stop the current topical application. Soak three times a day in warm water with soap. Start clindamycin, 300 mg three times a day for 10 days. Stop promptly if she has *diarrhea*. I will see her tomorrow.

Commentary: *purulent:* Infected. *diarrhea:* In this situation, an adverse effect of the medication, sometimes a sign of a potentially serious complication of the use of clindamycin.

Patient 24: J.L., Age 61

Headaches and hypertension: They persist. In addition, he has nausea from time to time. All of these symptoms are long-standing. On his own, he continues to take an over-the-counter preparation.

Exam: BP 120/80, P 60. Does not look acutely ill. Some limitation of rotation of neck to the left. Tenderness at *level of* C 4-5, left paravertebral area.

Continue atenolol 25 mg daily.

He wonders about referral to "neuropathologist" because of what he feels are "spasms of the blood vessels."

Head and neck ache may be due to cervical osteoarthritis. Get cervical spine x-rays. Add diazepam 2 mg #60, 1 four times a day. Return 2 weeks.

He has concerns about his wife, who has an ongoing sensation of "noise in her ears." He asks for her referral to the Mayo Clinic, and I suggest that she first return to her local ear specialist.

Commentary: *level of C4-5:* The back of the neck at the level of the fourth and fifth cervical vertebrae.

Patient 25: K.M., Age 67

Hypertension: no headaches or dizziness. Feels better on Vasotec than on Calan SR and is not "tired."

Exam: BP 160/70 sitting, 160/80 standing. P 80.

Increase Vasotec to 10 mg each a.m. Return in a month.

Diabetes: Blood sugar now is 257 at 2:50 p.m. Urged to lose weight.

Patient 26: L.N., Age 72 (Telephone)

Constipation: We discussed her bowel problem. Milk of magnesia taken 4 days a week seems to help. On the fifth day, she has some diarrhea. Change to milk of magnesia, 15-30 cc at bedtime as needed.

Some dizziness. Change diazepam to 2 mg four times a day, only as needed, instead of regularly four times a day.

Commentary: *Constipation:* Though often a trivial and passing symptom, constipation may be painful and disabling and needs to be addressed carefully. Sometimes constipation may be a symptom of a serious illness or an adverse side effect of medication.

Patient 27: M.O., Age 49

Edema, left leg: persists and is somewhat more prominent now, with some discomfort. He continues on anticoagulation.

Exam: BP 130/80, P 80. Does not look acutely ill. Gait is normal. Left leg: 2+ edema.

He has swelling that extends up into his thigh. No appreciable pelvic pain, but lymphatic obstruction needs to be considered.

Continue current regimen. Return 2 weeks.

Commentary: *Edema:* Abnormal accumulation of fluid, often graded qualitatively from 0 to 4+.

END OF THE DAY

At the end of the office day, I return to the hospital to see one of my patients for a second time. Then I go home to my family.

Patient 28: N.P., Age 40

In the evening, I receive a telephone call from the husband of a patient, a 40-year-old woman. He tells me, "She's talking and she's not making any sense." On the way to their home, I begin thinking about what might be wrong with her. (See Case 2 in chapter 10 for a discussion of this patient.)

I have presented twenty-eight separate transactions, a complex day filled with a variety of problems and decisions. A student or a patient could legitimately ask: "How do physicians manage such a day? How can we do it efficiently, make best use of the time, and give it some order? How do we gather and handle all the information and keep it all straight? How do we define the issues? When do we call a consultant? How do we choose the consultant? What do we do when we have no idea what is wrong with the patient? How do we avoid mistakes? How do we handle mistakes when we make them?

"Is the information we have important or trivial? When problem A occurs following problem B, did A cause B? Do all the present problems define the context of a new problem, or should we look elsewhere, beyond the confines of the identified problems?

"How can we let the patient know that we are aware of all the information, that the patient is the only person on our mind at the time? How can we make it easy for the patient to tell the story?

"How can we do all of this in a way that is satisfying not only for the patient, but also for us, the physicians? How do doctors integrate their personal and professional lives?"

The next chapters address these questions regarding what it is like to be a physician—and other questions too. Which considerations are universal to all patients? Which are unique to the individual patient? And where do we start?

We start with the history.

Chapter 9

The Medical History

"No two people tell a story the same way."

The ability to explore the patient's story and then transform it into a cohesive narrative from which decisions about diagnosis and treatment are made defines a good physician. When physicians interview a patient, they "take a history." When they write it down, they "record the history." When they inquire from a colleague about a patient's illness, they ask, "What's the history?" As a first step in diagnosis, taking the medical history is more important than the physical examination or any tests. Only on rare occasion—patients who are unconscious or otherwise unable to speak reliably in their own behalf, for instance—are the other elements more important.

Previously I described a five-step process in the medical transaction: the story, the history, the issues, the doctor-patient relationship, and, the final step, the question "What did I learn?" To the extent that the history, the edited and abbreviated version of the story, is accurate, valid, and complete, the issues will be comparably well defined. A sloppy history severely compromises the whole process.

This chapter describes ways physicians encourage patients to tell their stories, how doctors transform the stories into the "medical history," how the stories and the history become the basis for diagnosis and treatment, and how this whole process can run amok.

GENERAL HISTORY AND THE MEDICAL HISTORY

Insights from the study of history in general help us understand all the dimensions of the medical history. We speak of ancient history, modern history, and current history, of national history and local history, of cultural history, economic history and family history. There is reliable, corroborated history, and history that is unreliable—fantasized, self-serving, and uncorroborated.

What actually happened is the *story*. *History* is what was recorded. Good history is the sum of many moments, what led up to those moments, what took place thereafter, the consequences for those involved, and their reactions. History is not simply the account of the events; it is an integration of all that is germane into a coherent account. Without that information, we squander the opportunity to learn as much as we can *about* the events and *from* them. By exploring the story, we have the opportunity to tease out causes and contributing factors, nuances, and new insights. Story is fact. History, at its best, approximates fact, but it is also inference: Did one event cause another, or was it coincidence? *What can we learn?*

If the story is the whole truth, then history is really the story "as told to" or "as seen by" the historian and may represent only part of the truth. As the actual event becomes more remote from the time the historian investigates and records it, the account becomes less reliable. Complex events are more difficult to describe and validate, as are inferences from them. We enhance the quality of history by getting other points of view. Bias, prejudice, preconceptions of what happened, and ignorance of what might be important or when the story really started get in the way of good history.

It is no different with the medical history. If its purpose is to aid in the diagnosis and treatment, then we must gather all the information we can to help us in that task. Doing it well serves the patient, but it also maintains the physician's stance as a lifelong student, not simply learning *about* each patient, but also learning *from* each patient. How to develop the history, how to talk to people, and how to listen are all dimensions of the human side of medicine.

In the medical context, like history in general, "the story" is all that happened, and "the medical history" is the abbreviated, edited story. The story, by definition, is always the same. The history varies according to the skill, point of view, fund of knowledge, and perceptiveness of the physician. The credential of "physician" gives privileged access to the patient's story. In the process of taking the history, the patient is the eyewitness, and the physician is the detective; the patient, the speaker, the doctor, the listener; the patient, the narrator, the doctor, the recorder; the patient, the author, the doctor, the editor; the patient, the teacher, the doctor, the student. And so one of the ways to judge the skill and level of professional competence is the degree to which the physician is a detective, listener, recorder, editor, and student.

Specifically the medical history is the sum of

- The "chief complaint," in the patient's own words, what brought the patient to the doctor.
- The "history of the present illness," the details of the chief complaint.
- The "past history," details of previous illnesses and operations, medications, and allergies.
- The "family history," a listing of family members' important illnesses, which may put the patient at increased risk.
- The "psychosocial history," selected details of the patient's life story.
- The "review of systems," an inquiry into common symptoms related to each organ system.

Together they provide the physician context for the problem at hand, a "sense of history" similar to that which wise statespersons use as they approach a crisis. In this process, physicians question, listen, and amplify; interpret and validate; edit, compose, and record; critique and learn; and empathize and form a relationship. Each of these steps has potential for flaws, and so physicians need to do them well.

We question, listen, and amplify. For example,

Doctor: What brings you to the office? (This is called an "open-ended question," one that encourages the patient to tell a story. A "closed-ended question," such as "Do you smoke?" can be answered "yes" or "no.")

Patient: I've got pain in my stomach. (In the patient's own words, this becomes the chief complaint.)

D: Tell me about it.

P: Last night I didn't feel so well after supper, and I started to get this pain here, around my belly button. I didn't think too much about it, but the pain kept on. By the time I went to bed, it was a little worse, but I was able to sleep until about 6 this morning, when I woke up because the pain was worse yet. That's when I called you.

D: What else can you tell me about it?

P: I vomited just before I called you.

D: Had you ever had pain like this before? (A "closed-ended" question.)

P: No, this is the first time.

D: Where is the pain now?

P: (pointing to the lower right side of his abdomen) Down here.

D: When was your last bowel movement?

P: Yesterday morning.

D: Any blood in your urine?

And so on, with a series of open-ended questions, then more precise questions and refinements of the answers. This exchange is enough to create a strong suspicion of acute appendicitis. The story, told spontaneously, then followed by a few questions and then an examination, points toward the diagnosis. "I've got pain in my stomach" is too vague for a definitive diagnosis; the rest of the history-taking process helps to get the answer. We repeat this routine of questioning with each new problem.

We interpret. Patients tell their stories in their own "code" or manner of speaking. Only rarely does a patient declare, "I have appendicitis," and even then, if not validated with proper inquiry and documentation, it may be in error. The physician translates the story and "decodes" it.

We validate. We validate further by correlating one part of the story with another or with information from prior records, family, or close associates. To the extent that the history at hand does not accurately reflect the story, it is helpful to have that additional point of view. Sometimes a consultant helps.

We edit and compose. The medical history is more than a combination of words like "diabetes," "appendicitis," "pain," "chest pain," and "shortness of breath"; rather, it is an organized presentation of a great deal of information. If world history provides context to single moments in history, then the complete medical history provides the "clinical context" to the medical moment. Without knowing the context, physicians limit what they learn about the patient and from the patient.

Think of history in photographic terms. History is not a single snapshot; it is a movie, a sequence of snapshots, a story with a time dimension. We come into the movie during one short segment. If it is a mystery, the clues accumulate and the "solution" is clearer at the end. So it is with the medical history. Physicians enter at a certain moment. Early in the story, the solution may not be so clear; later, almost anyone could figure it out.

From an artist I learned, "No two people tell a story the same way."[1] Some ways are more effective than others. What the patient says is often a sequence of spontaneous, short narratives, connected haphazardly. As physicians, our task is to recognize the connections, apply order, make sense, clarify and separate the issues, and do it in a way that does not undermine or destroy the sense of the patient's story and cause us to draw the wrong conclusions and take inappropriate action. How well the doctor edits the story determines how useful the material is in leading to a diagnosis, treatment plan, and prognosis. Editing takes many forms: determining when the story actually began, what is important and what is superfluous, what are data and what are inferences, and when to quote the patient directly.

We record. The physician records the history of the above interview in this way:

This 44-year-old man comes to the office with the
    Chief complaint: "I've got pain in my stomach."
    History of the present illness: He was in good health about 7 p.m. yesterday, after supper, when he noticed periumbilical [the area around the "belly button"] pain, not especially severe, which persisted and slowly worsened. By this morning, 11 hours later, the pain was localized to the right lower quadrant of the abdomen. He vomited once, after the onset of the pain. He had a normal bowel movement yesterday and has had no hematuria [blood in the urine]. He has not had previous similar pain.

We critique. When we take and record the history, we discover gaps and new connections between events, and we look at ways to do it better. Whether the process of interviewing is good or bad can make a difference in the relationship with the patient and a difference in both the process of care and the outcome of the illness.

We learn. Our patients are our teachers. From their stories, we learn most of what we need to know about them and their diagnosis and how to question the next patient with a similar complaint.

We empathize and form a relationship. As physicians, it is our job to project ourselves into the story well enough to understand it and the patient and to express that understanding. The interaction demonstrates our interest, establishes a model for further transactions, and helps to establish or reinforce the relationship. The relationship facilitates care. We cannot do that with a questionnaire.

THE PSYCHOSOCIAL HISTORY

Attending to the psychosocial history recognizes what is going on in patients' lives as an important factor in how they feel. We learn how they deal with illness and other dilemmas and how they relate to others. It tells us *what it's like* to be the patient. Even in the absence of a psychological illness, the psychosocial history widens the physician's view and the context in which the illness occurs; a simple list of illnesses too narrowly defines the patient.

The physician explores the psychosocial history in various ways. She asks, "What's this illness been like for you?" She explores the symbolism of the illness by asking, "What does this mean to you?" Patients may respond: "My arthritis means I'll be disabled." "My high blood pressure? My father had high blood pressure and he died when he was 50." "I'm worried I have cancer."

Questions using the BATHE[2] technique help:

B Background	"What's going on in your life?"
A Affect (the feeling state)	"How do you feel about what is going on?"
T Trouble	"What about the situation troubles you the most?"
H Handle	"How do you handle that?"
E Empathy	Some statement of empathy that validates the patient's reflections and brings closure to this part of the inquiry, such as "That must have been very difficult for you."

Without this inquiry, the opportunity to help, not simply with a diagnosis, but also with advice about what is going on in the patient's life, is too limited. Stories of patients' illnesses come from broader stories of their lives, and remedies have to be compatible with that story. It is folly to propose treatment with an expensive blood pressure medicine, for instance, if the patient cannot afford the drug. It does not help to talk about limb amputation if the patient has decided that life is not worth living. In the story below, prescribing more physical therapy for this patient's back pain was not helpful; knowing more about his psychosocial history explained why his recovery from the injury had been slow.

For two years now, this 55-year-old butcher had persistent back pain, despite several careful physical examinations, multiple x-rays, and weeks of physical therapy and medication. A different physician questioned him more completely about his psychosocial history and learned that he had been a butcher for many years, happy in his work and well regarded. When a grocery chain took over his market, he felt devalued in his new position, simply one of many other employees. After a few months in his new job, he slipped and fell, striking his back. He had survived a concentration camp during the Holocaust, when prisoners were identified by a number tattooed on their forearms. "How did this new job make you feel?" his physician asked. His answer was the key to a larger story: "Like a number."

TEACHING THE MEDICAL HISTORY PROCESS

To the extent that the process of taking and recording the clinical history is faulty and the psychosocial context is ignored, subsequent diagnostic and therapeutic action can be misdirected or incomplete, and appropriate care can be delayed—or never provided. It is critical that physicians-in-training learn good, reproducible, and valid techniques early in their careers.

How do we interview patients and get them to tell their stories? How do we teach this skill? The physician-teacher models the process. To illustrate these techniques, I use a videotaped interview of a patient with metastatic colon cancer. I explain the structure of the interview before I play the tape. My questions will be open-ended initially, I tell the students, and I will allow her to tell her story at her own pace, without interruption. During that time, I will make only a few notes. When she is through with her spontaneous narrative, I will go back over the story with her and ask questions to clarify and amplify what she has told me. I will draw on my experience and my curiosity to come more precisely to a diagnosis or at least a "differential diagnosis" (see chapter 10) of what her problems are. During this time, I will also explore her understanding of her illness, her reaction to it, her ways of coping, and where she gets her moral and emotional support. I will use all of this information as I plan her treatment and, more broadly, how I will help to care for her. And throughout the whole interview, I will ask myself, "What did I learn?"

I teach these lessons.

- Trust your patients and believe their story. Only rarely are patients dishonest. Trust is a two-way street: Unless you trust them, they will not trust you.

- Remember, you are learning *about* the patient, and if you are doing it right, you will be learning *from* the patient. The patient is your teacher. One of my students wrote, "The conversation should be treated at first as a lecture, where the patient is the authority on her own condition and her body." You can start with little or no technical knowledge. A good way to develop this skill is to imagine that you are the first person ever to interview a person with colon cancer, appendicitis, diabetes, shortness of breath, or any other complaint or illness, that you are going to be the first ever to describe this illness, and that your patient is your only resource. Then allow the patient to tell his story.

- First ask open-ended questions, that is, questions allowing the patient to respond with a narrative. Start with, "What brings you here?" followed by "What was that like?" and "Tell me about it." Then listen and become fascinated by what the patient says and how. Reserve questions that can be answered "Yes" or "No" until the very end.

- Do not interrupt. Allow silence when it occurs. Silence may mean that the patient is thinking, trying to organize thoughts, perhaps struggling with a difficult emotion. Intruding on that silence may fracture the sequence of thoughts and feelings. Often what follows an uninterrupted silence may be valuable information.

- Review and revise. Tell the patient your understanding of the story. If one part of the story does not jibe with another, go over the inconsistencies.

- Regard the initial history as neither definitive nor final. Inquire about information the patient may have forgotten or hidden. If you are stuck on the diagnosis, go back and reinterview the patient. Sometimes the physician has neglected to explore an important part of the story. Sometimes the patient has forgotten to tell an important part or has not yet developed sufficient trust in the physician to reveal an especially sensitive bit of information.

- Ask this final question, "Is there any question I did not ask that I should have?"

- Learn from your cumulative experience. The more histories we take, the greater our intuition becomes after hearing but one sentence, such as "I had breast cancer in 1991." Beyond the diagnosis, we can imagine the shock of discovering the lump, the shattering experience of first hearing the diagnosis, the anticipation of the surgery and the anesthetic, the uncertainty, and the family's experience. "Her father was an alcoholic." "When she was 13, her parents divorced." "Twelve years ago, I had coronary bypass surgery." Even without the details, we know that these are dramatic moments and there is a complex story behind each statement. The story of a patient with coronary heart disease in chapter 1 illustrates this well.

WHAT CAN GO WRONG

The challenge is to consolidate and integrate the material from taking the history without destroying the essence of the story, in order to draw valid conclusions and take appropriate action. Sometimes physicians get in the way of a good medical history.

- We interrupt. Interrupting prematurely disrupts the story and the association of one element to another.

- We misunderstand. We hear things differently from how they were spoken. When two people disagree on the "facts," whether it is two professionals or a professional and a patient, it is usually because each has a different view or understanding of the patient's story. We must be certain that we are operating off the same story.

- We do not take enough time. We can misjudge people because we do not take the time.

- We miss the whole story by limiting the scope of the inquiry. Sometimes knowing the history from its beginning provides clues for preventing recurrence of the illness. A 40-year-old woman had abdominal pain following surgery for gallstones. Was the postoperative pain a consequence and complication of her surgery or part of the story that led up to the surgery and not even related to her gallstones? Did her marriage breakup have anything to do with the pain? Wise physicians look beyond the obvious events toward the real beginning of the story in order to draw the correct conclusions, fashion the best treatment, and learn the right lessons.

- We fail to recognize that it may take more than one interview to discover a key detail that will help in the diagnosis. Sometimes patients talk about their fears, addictions, or other sensitive matters only after a relationship is well established.

- There may be a "language barrier." The barrier may be as obvious as that between an English-speaking physician and a non-English-speaking patient. It may also be a metaphor for more subtle language difficulties, when a physician speaks in medical jargon.

When we fail to recognize the difference between primary data and inference, we unconsciously manufacture our own story with incomplete information, and we draw incorrect conclusions. Once, when I was an intern on the psychiatry service at Minneapolis General Hospital, the physicians, nurses, and social workers spent an inordinate amount of time speculating about why a patient wore sunglasses all the time. "He's hiding from us," they suggested. "He's turned inward. He's afraid of the 'light' of self-recognition." I finally asked the patient, "Why?" His response: "Because my other glasses are broken."

Describing his physician-hero, Robertson Davies wrote, "It also taught me a lesson about being a doctor: You can't really form an opinion about somebody until you have seen the place where they live."[3] I see this observation both in a literal sense and as an apt metaphor. If we literally cannot see "the place where they live," then we must try to visualize it. The medical interview and history-taking process are the best gateway to those insights.

There are many highs in medicine—diagnosing an elusive illness or preserving someone's life with complex, meticulous care in the midst of a potentially catastrophic illness. But these are rare occurrences compared with the more common and consistently exciting everyday transaction of "taking the history." There is a joy in gathering and using the information, gaining insights, probing the essence of a patient's life, and participating in the patient's drama.

From that starting point, physicians can then proceed to diagnosis and a plan of care and treatment.

Chapter 10

Diagnosis: How Physicians Reason

"A problem defined is a problem half solved."

A diagnosis dictates decisions and action. It can be a simple one, easy and quick to make: the common cold, sprained ankle, pneumonia, cystitis (bladder infection). Or it can be more complex, requiring substantial thought and time: bacterial endocarditis, a complex illness caused by a heart valve infection; ulcerative colitis, sometimes beginning as mild diarrhea instead of the more dramatic bloody bowel movements; dissecting aortic aneurysm, a tearing of the main artery leading from the heart and often mimicking the symptoms of a heart attack. A diagnosis, even a tentative one—the answer to the questions "What is wrong?" or "What is going on?"—allows the physician to make decisions and take action.

Like the medical history, diagnosis is an ongoing *process* of defining and refining the issues. It is not enough to declare, "She has coronary heart disease." Over and over, the physician needs to ask these questions:

- Can the diagnosis be refined further and more precisely? Different varieties of the same illness require different treatment.

- Does the diagnosis require urgent treatment? Delay in treatment may cause irreversible harm.

- Should I look for other illnesses associated with this one? One diagnosis may be the only clue to an associated illness that requires separate consideration and treatment.
- What psychological and social factors pertain? Some of those factors may clarify the diagnosis, and some diagnoses have substantial impact on the patient and the family.
- What else could this be? From an incorrect diagnosis, the physician will make invalid decisions about treatment and prognosis.

Our ability to describe the system we use to solve problems is important. This allows us to solve individual diagnostic and therapeutic problems consistently and efficiently, mature as problem solvers, and learn from our experience. Regardless of our store of knowledge, we are called upon to solve problems of such variety and complexity in the course of normal practice that we require a dependable problem-solving methodology to make best use of that knowledge and skill.

Physicians constantly build on experience. Experience with other patients helps us address the patient at hand. Knowing about other illnesses associated with a diagnosis, complications, beneficial and adverse reactions to drugs and other treatments, and psychosocial issues adds to the quality of the diagnostic process. All of this experience helps us understand, anticipate, and empathize.

DIFFERENTIAL DIAGNOSIS AND NAMING THE PROBLEM

What a physician does to make a diagnosis, a process called "differential diagnosis," begins by giving a problem a name and then exploring the possible diagnostic solutions to the problem. To introduce the students in my seminar to the process of diagnosis, we work together in class on this simple problem:

Case 1

One evening you are called at home by your patient, a 50-year-old man, who says, "I'm having pain in my stomach, low on the right side." As you are driving over to his home, you begin thinking about what might be wrong with him.

I suggest these questions to help them in their deliberations:
1. *What is the name of the problem?* I do not mean, "What is the diagnosis?" but rather, "What would you call the problem he described?" A problem name can certainly be a diagnosis, such as pneumonia, diabetes, or duodenal ulcer. Or the name can be a symptom, such as chest pain or shortness of breath. Name the problem as precisely as you can, I urge them, no more, no

less. To name the problem, one need not be medically sophisticated. "Headaches," "stomach cramps," "no pep," and "swollen knees" are part of everyone's vocabulary. The name of this man's problem is "right lower abdominal pain," but that is not enough to direct treatment, which could run the gamut from a heating pad for a sprained abdominal wall muscle to an operation for appendicitis. My goal is to teach the students the importance of how we name a problem. Giving a problem the wrong name and prematurely jumping to a diagnostic conclusion can delay treatment, bring about incorrect treatment, or imply a prognosis that may be either too optimistic or pessimistic. And certainly such an error can undermine the patient's future confidence in the skill of the physician.

2. *Where in the body is the disease?* What organs and structures are in this area? Even at the undergraduate level, most have a basic knowledge of human anatomy, and during the discussion, they acquire more. I ask them, "From front to back, what's in the right lower abdomen?" Any of these organs or tissues could have an abnormality that causes pain, I tell them.

3. On the basis of your answers to the previous questions and your own current knowledge, *what diagnoses might you consider as you try to answer the question, "What is wrong with this patient?"* What could be wrong with each of these organs or tissues? With very little prodding from me, they come up with this list:

Organ	The Students' List
Skin	Burn, cut
Muscle	Sprain
Small intestine	Ileitis
	Gastroenteritis
Large intestine	Colitis
	Cancer
Appendix	Appendicitis
Ureter	Kidney stone

4. The medical history is important. On the basis of your answer to the previous question, *what questions would you ask the patient that would help to clarify the nature of his illness and make a diagnosis?* What do you need to know to choose or eliminate each diagnosis you mention in question 3? Table 10.1 summarizes the process.

Each of these questions, though not definitive, moves the diagnostic process along. The presence of blood in the urine, for instance, along with inability of the patient to find a comfortable position would point toward a kidney stone. Weight loss over a period of weeks or longer might suggest co-

Table 10.1
Using the History as the First Step in the Differential Diagnosis of "Right
Lower Abdominal Pain" (in Case 1)

Organ	Disease or illness	Clarifying questions
Skin	Burn, cut	Have you injured or burned yourself?
Muscle	Sprain	Have you injured yourself?
Small intestine	Ileitis	Do you have diarrhea? Cramps? Have you lost weight? How long have you been ill?
	Gastroenteritis	Do you have diarrhea? Cramps? Does anyone in your family have a similar illness? How long have you been ill?
Large intestine	Colitis	Questions similar to above.
	Colon cancer	Have you lost weight? Have you had blood in your stools?
Appendix	Appendicitis	Have you been vomiting? Which came first, the pain or the vomiting? Have you lost your appetite?
Ureter	Kidney stone	Have you noticed blood in your urine? Can you find a comfortable position in which you have no pain?

lon cancer, ileitis, or colitis. If the person is younger, it is less likely that
cancer is the diagnosis.

It is not hard to see that a problem name may have many different solutions. Pain in the lower right side of the abdomen is often a symptom of appendicitis, but not always. The initial symptoms of a problem may be
different in different people. A patient with colon cancer may notice pain
as an initial symptom, or blood in the stool, or weight loss. Our diagnostic
skills become more refined as our knowledge and experience increase.
Naming the problem is important because it helps to define the additional
questions, the additional data that need to be accumulated, and the fund of
knowledge we need to approach a problem thoroughly. A problem defined
is a problem half solved.

With the lessons learned from Case 1, the class turns to a more difficult
diagnostic problem, a real one from my own experience (Patient 28, N.P.,
from chapter 8).

Case 2

In the evening, I receive a telephone call from the husband of a patient, a 40-year-old woman. He tells me, "She's talking and she's not making any sense." On the way to their home, I begin thinking about what might be wrong with her.

Together the students and I go through the same process.

1. *What is the name of the problem?* Here are some of their answers and my comments.

- "Brain tumor." Too precise, given the information provided. Though that may be the answer ultimately, the data do not warrant it just yet. The method of getting to the answer is important in order to be more consistently correct.
- "Not making any sense." Not a very technical answer, but not bad. At least it shows me where the student really is in his reasoning and where I need to start my teaching.
- "Confusion." Not bad either. Like "not making any sense," it allows for a thoughtful differential diagnosis, so long as each name prods the student into asking, "What are the possible causes?"
- "Dementia." Dementia is a permanent state, and her illness just began. Delirium, a more temporary state, may be a more appropriate term. Each of the terms, delirium and dementia, has its own differential diagnosis.
- "Change in mental status." We settle on this name for it is broad enough to lead to a productive diagnostic process and it does not prematurely restrict the choices.

2. *Where in the body is the disease?* The brain is the obvious answer. What organs, tissues, etc, are in this area? Nerve tissue, arteries, veins, blood. What does the brain need in order to function? Blood, oxygen, and glucose, for starters.

Then I introduce a nuance of the above question: *What other organs or organ systems of the body might contribute to the patient's problems? In what ways might they contribute?* By now, the students feel authorized to think more originally, broadly, and creatively. They add other items to their list:

- The circulatory system. The heart, if injured, may not be able to pump blood and glucose to the brain. Narrowed or completely blocked arteries may prevent adequate blood and glucose flow.
- The respiratory system: In the presence of diseased lungs, the supply of oxygen may be limited and the ability to rid the body of carbon dioxide may be impaired.

- The pancreas: The pancreas could be producing too much insulin, lowering the blood sugar level and altering brain function.

3. *On the basis of your answers to the previous questions and your own current knowledge, what diagnoses might you consider as you try to answer the question, "What is wrong with this patient?"*
Again, we start by organs.

- The brain: stroke, tumor, subdural hematoma (a blood clot usually following trauma), psychological issues.
- The heart: myocardial infarction (heart attack), congestive heart failure.
- The arteries: carotid artery stenosis (narrowing of the artery from cholesterol deposits).
- The lungs: pneumonia, pulmonary embolus (a blood clot formed elsewhere and lodged in the lung).
- The pancreas: insulinoma (a tumor that secretes too much insulin).

Then we enlarge the list as we go beyond the confines of organs and organ systems. What about drug-induced illness from prescribed drugs? If the patient has diabetes and takes insulin, maybe her blood sugar level is too low. If the patient takes a diuretic medication for heart failure or hypertension, and especially if she has been sweating a lot, maybe the blood sodium concentration is sufficiently diminished to cause a change in mental status. What about illness from nonprescribed drugs—alcohol, marijuana, others? What about toxins? What else?

4. *What questions would you ask that would help to clarify the nature of her illness and make a diagnosis?* Table 10.2 summarizes the process.
So that the students begin to understand not only the technical aspects of the clinical drama but also the human, psychosocial parts, I ask them, "What do you think this experience is like for her and her family? What do you think this experience is like for the physician?"
Studying the case this way presents many "teachable moments," opportunities for students to learn about what physicians do, how they do it in a reproducible fashion, the differential diagnosis of "change in mental status," some of the symptoms of heart attack, pneumonia, stroke, and hypoglycemia, and what all of this is like for the patient, the family, and the doctor.

Table 10.2
Using the History as the First Step in the Differential Diagnosis of "Change in Mental Status" (in Case 2)

Organ/origin	Disease or illness	Clarifying questions
Brain	Stroke	How did this begin—suddenly or gradually?
	Tumor	How did this begin—suddenly or gradually?
	Subdural hematoma	Have you struck your head?
	Psychological issues	What's going on in your life?
Heart	Myocardial infarct	Have you had pain in your chest?
	Congestive heart failure	Have you been short of breath? Do your ankles swell?
Lungs	Pneumonia	Have you had a cough or fever?
	Pulmonary embolus	Have you been short of breath? Have you had pain in your chest?
Pancreas	Insulin-secreting tumor	Has this ever happened before? If so, what part of the day does it happen?
	Diabetes mellitus	Do you have diabetes? Do you take medicine for it? When did you last eat?
Toxins		Are you exposed to anything potentially toxic at home or at work?
Drugs		How much do you drink? When did you take your last drink? Do you use other drugs?

LOOKING AT THE RELATIONSHIP BETWEEN PROBLEMS: THE CLINICAL CONTEXT AND THE PROBLEM-ORIENTED SYSTEM

Naming problems and writing them down allows the physician to study the relationships of one to the others, ponder possible causes and effects, consider the validity of past diagnoses and the effectiveness of past treatment, and arrive at a solution to each new problem that makes complete use of all the information available. Beyond the fact that this exercise in precision, completeness, and evaluation tends to expose more information on each patient than we could otherwise get, a list of problems provides us with an extra dimension in problem solving, the *clinical context*.

For instance, examining the relationship between "abdominal pain" and "diabetes mellitus" stimulates the student to ask: "Does their coexistence in the same patient alter the way I look at each one of them? Does appendicitis have different symptoms and manifestations in patients with diabetes? Are there special considerations in the differential diagnosis of abdominal pain present in the patient with diabetes? Are special therapeutic considerations necessary in caring for the patient with diabetes who has appendicitis? What is it like for a patient who has diabetes and then develops appendicitis?"

Naming the problem, looking at the relationship between problems, taking advantage of each teachable moment, learning from experience, and identifying gaps in our knowledge come together in the *problem-oriented system*,[1] a technique that is technologically simple and yet very, very sophisticated.

I use the following history, a fictitious case, to illustrate how the system works. I integrate into it a series of tasks and questions for the students, and I direct them to construct a *problem list* and then use the list to identify the issues, make clinical decisions about diagnosis and treatment, discover possible relationships between the problems and their treatments, and teach themselves. I provide additional information, help them formulate the questions, facilitate the discussion, validate their techniques and conclusions, and provide a model for reasoning.

Case 3

S.M., age 73, is hospitalized because of diabetes, out of control, on 12/10/98.

Diabetes mellitus was first diagnosed in 1965 when she rapidly lost weight. Blood sugar at that time was 520, a very high concentration. Over the years she has been treated with insulin and currently self-administers NPH insulin 30 units each morning. (NPH insulin may have its maximum effect on the blood sugar level about eight hours after it has been administered, and so a common time for a person to have a period of hypoglycemia [low blood sugar or insulin reaction] after a morning injection is late in the afternoon.) Her admission this time is precipitated by nausea. On admission, she is dehydrated, and blood chemistry determinations confirm the presence of diabetic ketoacidosis (a complex disorder of body chemistry, affecting the concentration of water, sugar, sodium, potassium, and products of metabolism). She is treated with extra insulin and intravenous fluids and by the time of discharge a week later is feeling well, and diabetes is well controlled on a 2,000-calorie diabetic diet and NPH insulin 35 units daily.

Cerebral arteriosclerosis was diagnosed in 1990 following a stroke that left her right arm and leg weak. She had no recurrence. Occasionally she has become confused.

She had a duodenal ulcer in 1990 at which time she complained of heartburn. X-rays of her stomach and duodenum confirmed the diagnosis. She has no current symptoms.

She has been depressed in the past and was hospitalized in 1992 for three months, during which time she received electroconvulsive therapy (shock therapy).

Twenty-four years ago, she developed hives after an injection of penicillin.

She is a widow, lives alone, and rarely sees her two daughters.

The students follow these steps.

1. *Construct a problem list*, dating the onset of each problem as precisely as possible.

This is their initial list.

1. Diabetes mellitus, onset 1965
2. Nausea, onset 12/10/98
3. Dehydration, onset 12/10/98
4. Diabetic ketoacidosis, onset 12/10/98

We then talk about the different causes of nausea. In this case, I tell them that the nausea and the dehydration are part of the clinical picture of diabetic ketoacidosis. We then revise and consolidate the first four problems into one:

1. Diabetes mellitus, onset 1965
   A. Diabetic ketoacidosis, onset 12/10/98

and complete the list as follows:

2. Cerebral arteriosclerosis, onset 1990
   A. Stroke (weakness, right arm and leg), onset 1990
3. Duodenal ulcer, onset 1990
4. Depression, onset 1993
5. Penicillin allergy (hives), onset 1974

Following discharge from the hospital on 12/17/98, she returns home. One week later, on 12/24/98, she is readmitted to the hospital because of nausea, and again her diabetes is found to be out of control. After three days, diabetes is again well controlled on NPH insulin 35 units a day and a 2,000-calorie diabetic diet. On 12/30/98, about 4 p.m., she becomes irritable and makes romantic advances to an orderly half her age. This is unusual behavior for her.

2. Name the new problem and add it to the problem list. Regardless of the magnitude or duration of the problem, give it a name. Failing to identify and name problems, one is apt to miss diagnostic clues of crucial importance. There are actually two new problems: (1) a repeat episode of diabetic ketoacidosis, which is added to the list as a second event:

1. Diabetes mellitus, onset 1965
   A.   Diabetic ketoacidosis, onset 12/10/98, <u>12/24/98</u>

and (2) the episode occurring about 4 p.m. I ask, "What is this episode? How shall we name it?" The students come up with these more or less sophisticated names: irritable, romantic advances, confusion, insulin reaction, and change in mental status. As in Case 2, we choose the name that allows the broadest inquiry, "change in mental status," and add it to the list.

1. Diabetes mellitus, onset 1965
   A.   Diabetic ketoacidosis, onset 12/10/98, 12/24/98
2. Cerebral arteriosclerosis, onset 1990
   A.   Stroke (weak right arm and leg) 1990
3. Duodenal ulcer, onset 1990
4. Depression, onset 1993
5. Penicillin allergy (hives), onset 1974
6. Change in mental status, onset 4 p.m., 12/30/98

3. Address the possible diagnostic solutions to the new problem by scanning the problem list and asking: "Is the new problem related to any of the other problems? Is the new problem related to the treatment of any other problems?" The differential diagnosis of "change in mental status" differs in this patient from Case 2 because the clinical context is different. Each element of this inquiry is an opportunity to teach about each of the diseases and supplement the student's fund of knowledge, using the problem list as a reference point. Table 10.3 summarizes the process.

4. Make a diagnosis. Collect additional information from the history, physical examination and laboratory data.

Table 10.3
Differential Diagnosis of "Change in Mental Status" (in Case 3)

Problem	Related to the problem	Related to the treatment of the problem	Action
Diabetes mellitus	Hyperglycemia (high blood sugar) can cause change in mental status	Hypoglycemia (low blood sugar) can cause change in mental status.	Immediately give glucose. (Since hypoglycemia requires immediate treatment, and no harm can be done by treating it with glucose even if this is not the cause, do this first and quickly.) Check blood sugar concentration.
Cerebral arteriosclerosis	She could be having another stroke.	She is on no medication for this problem.	Examine for other signs of stroke.
Duodenal ulcer	She could be bleeding from an ulcer. (Bleeding may lower blood pressure and diminish circulation to the brain, causing change in mental status.)	She is on no medication for this problem.	Check the blood pressure; check for other signs of blood loss.
Depression	She could be more depressed.	She is on no medication for this problem.	Interview her for possible clues to depression. Ask, "Are you depressed?"
Penicillin allergy	An allergic reaction can cause changes in mental status. Unless she has been given penicillin inadvertently, this is an unlikely cause.		

5. *Implement therapy.* Especially consider what immediate therapeutic step should be taken. As indicated above, the urgent action is to treat the possible hypoglycemic reaction. Had her action, "making romantic advances to an orderly half her age," been dismissed as unimportant, the physician and the nurse would have overlooked and left untreated the easily treated insulin reaction, a medical emergency.

She is discharged on 1/2/99 on a 2,000-calorie diabetic diet and NPH insulin 35 units daily. On 1/9/99 she is readmitted because of nausea, and again diabetes is out of control.

6. *What is going on?* This is now the third time that the patient has been hospitalized with a similar illness, diabetic ketoacidosis, following adequate control on a routine that involves the same diet and the same dose of insulin. Any problem that recurs frequently requires a special inquiry.

We revise the problem statement:

1. Diabetes mellitus, onset 1965
   A. Diabetic ketoacidosis onset 12/10/98, 12/24/98, 1/2/99 (<u>a recurrent problem</u>)

When I ask the students, "What is going on?" I mean, "Why is this problem recurring?"—another teachable moment. Unless we recognize that a recurrent problem requires a separate inquiry, we will fail to address important issues separate from the basic diagnosis. The students speculate and recognize that psychosocial matters often have real importance. She may not be following her diet because she is depressed and wants to die, because she is alone, lonely, and craves attention, or because she cannot afford the special foods. She may not be taking her insulin correctly because she cannot afford the medicine, the syringes, and the testing material. In addition, I point out that among the possible long-term effects of diabetes are visual problems and neuropathy (various disorders of the nervous system). Maybe she cannot see the insulin syringe because of the eye problems; maybe she no longer has the dexterity to manipulate the syringe because of the neuropathy.

Physicians learn in many ways: interactions with colleagues and patients, reading, attending lectures, seminars, and postgraduate courses. When we approach our work systematically, we are better able to learn from a primary source, our own experience, and move on more confidently to treatment and prognosis.

Chapter 11

Treatment and Prognosis

"First do no harm."

If all treatment were simple and without potentially adverse effects, decisions about treatment would be easy. For example:

- The treatment for an upper respiratory infection, the common cold, is nothing more than some medicine for comfort. Untreated, the patient may be uncomfortable for a few days, but she will suffer no long-term adverse effects.

- The treatment for a strep throat is penicillin. Untreated, the patient may develop rheumatic fever or glomerulonephritis, an inflammation of the kidney.

- The treatment for a skin laceration is sewing it up. Unsutured, it will heal poorly and may become infected.

- The treatment for appendicitis is appendectomy, usually a simple operation of low risk. There are no good alternatives. Anything other than appendectomy may lead to serious complications and premature death.

- The treatment for a compound fracture of the femur, where the bone fragments have broken through the skin, is reparative surgery. The choice is usually simple for the patient and the patient's family, for untreated, the fracture will be unstable and the patient will develop a severe life-threatening infection.

The treatment for S.M., Case 3 in chapter 10, is more complex, for there are many problems to consider concurrently. For the patient with coronary heart disease in chapter 1, the issues are complex also. Recall this part:

The next day the surgeon arrived and said that surgery *was* an option and that he could do it. With the cardiologist, I examined my choices. Treatment with medicine alone would not improve the long-term outlook. Angioplasty, using a balloon-tipped catheter to enlarge the areas of narrowing, might be a possible remedy but had its risks. Surgery, though also risky, seemed the best choice.

Most of the time, there are several treatment choices to consider in a patient with significant coronary artery disease: medication, bypass surgery, angioplasty, or combinations of them. Medication alone is least traumatic. Angioplasty, with or without a stent (a supporting structure inserted in the angioplasty site), often involves no more recovery time than that required for the angiogram. Bypass surgery is by far the most traumatic, for it involves surgery and anesthesia, a long recovery period, and potential complications of the surgery. All three, alone or in combination, may fail. The arteries treated with angioplasty or bypass may close, and drugs may be ineffective. Then how do we decide about treatment? What enters into the decision? Not all turns out well, and a primary value in medicine is, "First do no harm."

Consider first the treatment and the options available for this patient. The cardiologist decides about the best treatment by considering the outcome and the risks of treatment. He asks himself, "What is the course of this illness, coronary heart disease, with the patient's specific coronary artery anatomy, treated and untreated? What are the benefits and risks of treatment?" A good physician applies these questions to every treatment decision. Defining and *declaring* the prognosis have importance to the physician and to the patient. Unless both are convinced that the treatment will improve the outcome, there is no good reason to choose it.

A more precise way of framing the cardiologist's question is: "On the basis of the coronary artery anatomy, how much muscle would be injured were he actually to have a heart attack?" If the amount of muscle at risk is small, usually when only a small branch of a major artery is narrowed, then the risk of surgery or angioplasty is unwarranted, and medication is the best choice. But suppose the affected artery is a major one, serving a large volume of heart muscle. Then the choices may be different: angioplasty or bypass surgery. The technical details of the procedure enter into the choice between the two; some are best handled by one or the other.

Sometimes a "trial of therapy" serves as a method of diagnosis. For example:

- A confused patient who has diabetes and takes insulin may be given a glucose injection without a confirmatory blood sugar test if hypoglycemia is suspected. If the confusion clears promptly, then hypoglycemia is the likely cause of the confusion.

- A patient with episodes of chest pain may be given nitroglycerin. If the pain is relieved promptly, he may have angina.

- A patient with hoarseness may be told to "take aspirin, gargle with salt water, and call me in three days if you're no better." If the hoarseness has resolved, the symptom requires no further investigation. If it persists, the physician must look for serious causes.

Prognosis, the prediction of outcome, affects the choice of treatment, but that is not all. Anyone who has been through a difficult illness knows that the *process* of care is an important dimension of the treatment. To the patient with heart disease and to his wife (chapter 1), the cardiologist said, "Here is what I think and here is how I think we should proceed." Then he defined for them the issues and the coronary artery abnormalities, described the choices and potential benefits of each, explained that there were risks to each and also risks of doing nothing, and provided opportunity for questions. Having outlined the choices, he said, "Here is what I think is the best choice." He expressed his understanding and empathy, "I know that this is a lot to absorb all at once. What are your thoughts?"

He did not say, "Here are the choices, take your pick," because most patients are unable to make such complex choices without the physician's wisdom. While most patients will ultimately participate in the decision, it is the physician's responsibility to provide sufficient information and explanation, weight the choices on the basis of his knowledge and cumulative experience, and then make a recommendation.

Then there is the human side. Which treatment is best also has to do with the patient's values. Consider the case of the 75-year-old patient with major narrowing of his carotid artery. When his physician urged him to have surgery to lessen the risk of stroke, she also told him that the surgery itself could precipitate a stroke, though that was less likely. The patient said, "I've lived a good life. I'm ready to die. I'll take my chances without surgery."

The treatment choice also has to do with the patient's experience. What may seem like an obvious, easy choice to the physician may be unacceptable to the patient, who fears hospitalization or has a friend whose outcome from similar treatment was poor. "No, thanks!" was the patient's response to her physician who suggested back surgery for a ruptured disc. "My friend had that surgery and hasn't been able to walk since." "No, thanks!" was another patient's response to a proposal for chemotherapy for breast cancer. "I

don't want to lose my hair. I don't want to spend my last months vomiting."
Inquiring about that patient's experience and her knowledge of other patients' stories provided the opportunity for the physician and the patient to
talk further and reach a more informed decision. Cost may influence the
patient's decision. If the patient can afford neither the cost of treatment
nor its follow-up visits and tests, she may decline.

The physician's own experiences often influence what she recommends.
If, despite the statistics, the physician has had a bad experience using a specific drug or treatment, she will be reluctant to recommend it. For the physician, the important step is to identify all the issues in the use of a specific
treatment: Was the adverse effect even rarer when seen in its broader community use? Did it happen because it was used inappropriately?

Most decisions regarding diagnosis and treatment are simple. Those that
deal with several concurrent illnesses and treatments are more difficult.
The more complex the illness, the greater the likelihood that the physician
will need help from others, for medicine is a collaborative profession, the
subject of the next chapter.

Chapter 12

Medicine Is a Collaborative Profession

"Know your resources."

Most of medical practice is straightforward, enabling a former Gloucester associate to observe years ago: "Ninety percent of what one needs to know in medicine is within the ken of 90 percent of the doctors." For that which is not, we turn to others. Medicine is a collaborative profession. We cannot do it alone.

Only after a few years in practice did I begin to recognize the true meaning of "collaboration" and "the clinical professions." Until then, I thought that doctors consulted only with doctors, nurses with nurses, etc. Now I know better. "The clinical professions" include everyone who is professionally trained to care for people: physicians, nurses, social workers, clergy, and therapists of all kinds. What is especially fascinating is how our professional paradigms and needs overlap and how much we can teach each other about the care of our patients.[1] Much of that overlap lies in the human side of medicine.

The collaboration between nurse and physician has been around a long time; each is an extension of the other. Especially in recent years in the hospital, home, and nursing home, nurses and doctors have become partners, extending each others' insights and observations. Wise nurses and doctors ask of each other, "What do you need to know from me that will help in the care of our patient?" Physicians have long underutilized the collaboration with social workers, who have skills in exploring and coordinating community resources and special talents in dealing with complex family relationships. Collaboration with hospital chaplains and other clergy provides additional views into the spiritual life and resources of the patient and family. Information from mental health professionals, physical and occupational therapists, and others in health care settings often holds the key to better care. The clinical professions have much to learn from each other.

Collaboration is "the ability to engage diverse groups in shared acts of discovery and evaluation."[2] No physician should be reluctant to ask for consultation if it will benefit the patient. Deciding which consultant to ask requires these sorts of considerations: How will the new information affect the decisions? Who is the best consultant for this problem and the patient? "When I chose you as a doctor, I also chose those doctors who are your consultants" was one patient's way of telling me that he approved of the urologist I had chosen to do his cancer surgery. He appreciated the urologist's technical skill, compassion, and understanding. He trusted the consultant because he trusted me. Through the years I discarded from my list of consultants those who were technically competent but incapable of developing an effective relationship with my patients.

Physicians consult with other physicians for various reasons.

- The consultant may have certain specific skills. The skills may be with procedures—gastroscopy or heart surgery, for example. They may be intellectual skills—expertise in diagnosing complex infections, for instance, or talent in diagnosing relatively rare illnesses with which few physicians have experience. A physician may ask for consultation because the consultant has therapeutic skills beyond his own—skill in using a drug or doing psychotherapy.

- It may be unclear what is going on. Consultation affords another way of looking at things.

- The physician may initiate consultation in order to validate her own views. She reflects, "I think I've got this right, but I'd like to bounce my ideas off a colleague whose opinion I trust." Like the patient noted before, even the physician "must visit a wise man from time to time to discover what one already knows."[3] Consultation provides an opportunity for self-critique.

- The physician may initiate consultation in order to reinforce for the patient and the family the physician's own approach, to validate for them the diagnosis, treatment, or prognosis. Sometimes the reputation of the consultant or the institution may be the reason. Even though the primary physician knows that the diagnosis is correct and that he has considered all the therapeutic options and chosen the best one, he recognizes that the patient may need the endorsement of the medical center or physician regarded as the best.

- The patient or the family may ask for consultation. Especially when things are not going well, consultation may reassure the family that "everything is being done." No physician should feel defensive when asked. A savvy cardiologist put the parents of a newborn son with a birth defect at ease when they requested another opinion: "We get others' opinions all the time. If you're wrong, you learn something; if you're right, you're a hero."

- Sometimes it is the personality. There may be conflicts between the patient and the physician that are unrelated to the medical issues at hand. Inserting another person into the transaction may resolve the conflict.

The level of consultation varies. There is the "formal consultation" and the "curbstone consultation." There is the focused consultation and a broader one. There is the single-visit consultation and an ongoing one, a series of meetings with the patient. And there is another kind, what I like to call the "self-consultation."

A *formal consultation* often takes this pattern.

- Surgeon to internist: "My patient is running a fever several days after his gallbladder surgery, and I can't find the cause. I'd like you to see him."

- Internist to another internist: "My patient has been tired now for several months, I've struggled to come up with an answer, and I've done a number of tests that haven't helped. I think she needs another point of view, and I'd like you to see her."

In the *curbstone consultation*, one physician asks another to help answer a question without seeing the patient.

- Internist to cardiologist: "I'm having trouble controlling my patient's arrhythmia (irregular heartbeat). What are your suggestions?"

- Cardiologist's response: "What's the clinical context for the arrhythmia? What else is going on with your patient?" She then suggests either that the dose of the drug be increased, that the current drug be changed, or that the patient does not need treatment because the arrhythmia is not dangerous and will cause neither symptoms nor shortening of life.

The "curbstone" may turn into a "formal" consultation when the cardiologist suggests that "there are enough unanswered questions and undefined issues that maybe I should see the patient."

The *focused consultation* addresses a single problem.

- Family physician to urologist: "Please see my patient with a kidney stone and help in her management."

- Internist to podiatrist: "Please see my patient who has diabetes and an ingrown toenail and do what needs to be done."

The *broad consultation* addresses many problems.

- Psychiatrist to internist: "My elderly patient is depressed. I'd like to know if there are any physical causes for her depression and I'd like you to help in her overall care."
- Surgeon to internist: "My patient is to have surgery next week for colon cancer. He needs an overall evaluation, and I'd like you to follow him in the hospital. See him as often as you think it's necessary, after he's had the surgery."

Sometimes what starts out one way changes to another. A request to focus on the care of diabetes turns into broader care and defining new issues, as in Case 2, in chapter 2. A curbstone consultation turns into a formal one. What seems to require only a single transaction turns into a series of meetings. Sometimes the wrong question is asked. Sometimes when the need warrants, the consultant does even more than asked.

Then there is the *self-consultation*. When I have been stymied over a patient's diagnosis or treatment, before I ask for consultation from a colleague, I will sometimes ask myself, "How would I approach this patient (or case or problem) if *I* were called to see him as a consultant?" I look at the case in a fresh way, reinterview the patient, review the patient's chart, reconstruct a problem list, define the issues afresh, and, often as not, come up with the elusive answers. When I do that, I achieve one of the goals of a good medical education: I become my own teacher.

The ideal consultation is one with give-and-take between the consultant and the referring physician, who may recall small nuances of the patient's history of importance to clinical decisions. The conversation provides the basis for a more complete and thorough consultation as physicians test each other's hypotheses and plans and raise questions the other had not thought about.

We ask for consultation when cases are complex. Certain illnesses have many issues with which to deal regarding cause, treatment, and a clinical course with many ups and downs. "Complicated cases are complicated," an orthopedist taught me, and acknowledging this reality helps to mobilize all the available resources. Complicated cases with many consultants work best when each knows who has the responsibility for what part of the patient's care. "Each one understood his role and the other's."[4] In addition, someone has to be in charge, a physician who acts as a "general contractor," the overseer of the process, and the interpreter and final common pathway to the patient and family. That person integrates all of the information, judges its worth, says "yes" or "no" to tests, procedures, and treatment, and helps to resolve conflicting points of view.

When no one is in charge, many things can go wrong. Ten years after a 70-year-old woman had a cystectomy (removal of the urinary bladder) for cancer, she began having fever, presumably from a kidney infection. Her consultants included a urologist and an infectious disease specialist. Treatment included surgical drainage of the kidney and intravenous antibiotics. Yet the fever persisted. The infectious disease specialist said, "If I could get the tube out, the fever would be gone." The urologist said, "She's getting better and can go home." Her daughter said, "She's worse. I'd like another opinion." Paying attention to the daughter's view, a new consultant, now in charge of the care, reinterpreted all the information and found the answer, unfortunately a recurrence of cancer, sometimes the cause of unexplained fever.

Sometimes the patient self-refers to the wrong consultant. Then it is the consultant's task to see that the patient gets to the right one or back to the primary doctor. When a 60-year-old woman saw an allergist to get skin tests for "asthma," he realized that her wheezing was not from asthma but rather from congestive heart failure and arranged for her internist to see her immediately.

For some patients, the mechanism of referral requires extra sensitivity. Referral to a mental health professional, for instance, often carries a stigma that can be overcome by the referring physician: "Just as I would call a surgeon if you had appendicitis because I don't have surgical skills, now I'm suggesting that I arrange for psychiatric consultation for similar reasons. I want you to be in the best hands possible, so that you can get better as quickly as possible. And during this time, I will continue to stay involved." A referral to an oncologist carries different burdens, for one is placing a patient with a life-threatening illness in another's hands.

The lessons from these examples apply to almost every consultation: the need for one physician to oversee and coordinate the care, the reassurance that the doctor will not abandon the patient, an adequate explanation for the referral, and the reassurance that the consultation will provide more, not less, than the patient is already getting. Even the expert consultant is not always right.

Patients and families are part of the collaboration process. I learned from a patient with breast cancer, "Cancer follows certain patterns, but its specifics are your own adventure." My 90-year-old friend and patient wisely declared, "I am the professor of myself." The patient's story provides the clues to diagnosis, and once a tentative diagnosis is made, further discussion with the patient helps to validate or refine the diagnosis. I will often say to a patient, "You've been ill for several months now. Surely you must have thought about what might be wrong with you." That conversation often flushes out more details. Patients and their families know the unique ways a disease behaves for them.

The "textbook" description of an insulin reaction is sweating, rapid heartbeat, and hunger; so when my patient with diabetes seemed especially surly after his leg surgery, I did not give it a second thought and said to his wife, "He seems to be behaving like his old self." She disagreed: "He's having an insulin reaction!" Her special knowledge of her husband prompted immediate treatment. Especially with diabetes, but also with other chronic illnesses, patients need to be their own consultant, because they need to make daily judgments. Part of our task as physicians is to reinforce that role as they address questions such as "If I'm going to be more active today, do I need to take less insulin? My toe looks red; do I need to see the doctor to check about infection?"

If not for dedicated family and friends, many patients would not survive. "Last summer my husband almost died [from knee surgery and a complicating infection]," one of my patients told me, "and we nursed him back to health." It is sometimes folly for a physician to tell a patient "You'll be well in X days, weeks, or months" or "You have three months to live," for people differ and patients know their strengths and resources better than the doctor.

TEACHING COLLABORATION

At the beginning of the course, I tell my students, "Though I want your papers to be your own work, I want you to get together with a class partner to talk it over before you begin to write. When you do this, you will clarify your ideas and identify gaps in your knowledge. You will recognize your prejudices and help each other to neutralize them. There is another reason to work with a partner: I want to emphasize to you that medicine is a collaborative profession. By working with a partner, you will get handy with that process and begin to discover the qualities of a good consultant as you and your partner teach each other and hone your skills."

In a class session on collaboration, we explore ways in which various clinical professionals work together and involve the patient and family. Social workers, public health nurses, and hospital chaplains help clarify and enlarge the story and the clinical history, identify the issues, and show how the relationship with the patients and their families can facilitate care. I encourage the students to review the case history before class and give some thought to the issues so that they can more fully participate in the discussion. As in a real situation, planning a patient-centered conference ahead of time rather than doing it at a moment's notice allows all of the participants the opportunity to organize their thoughts and questions and to focus more precisely.

One case we discussed was that of a 73-year-old man, whose dementia began subtly with slight memory difficulty and progressed over four years to confusion, loss of mobility, and incontinence. During that time, he had tests to check for treatable causes of his brain disorder and saw a neurologist. His internist shepherded him and his wife through this illness and ultimate admission to a nursing home, where he died.

During the class, the physician, social worker, nurse, chaplain, and the patient's widow had a conversation. We asked questions of each other, filled in the blanks of the history, got a further sense of the patient's and his wife's experience, and discovered where the care might have run amok. We defined the issues: What is the diagnosis? Is it treatable? What is the natural history of the illness? Where are the uncertainties? How are they coping with the illness? What are the implications regarding nursing home care? What are the losses? We considered the impact of his illness on the patient *and* his family, the need to provide care for both, the importance of addressing the psychological and social issues in his illness, and ways in which the patient, the family, the physicians, and other professionals could collaborate. We explored what we could learn from this story that has application to other patients and their illnesses.

We learned that separation, relief, guilt, and financial cost are among a family's concerns; that losses include independence, companionship, emotional support, and dignity; and that patients and their families fear a long illness that is "out of our control," with invasive tubes and other uncomfortable treatments. We learned the danger of making invalid assumptions, the need to respect the patient's right to take some risks, the importance of providing a safe environment for people to express themselves, and the need for someone to oversee the overall care.

We discovered that complex family relationships and conflicts become more evident at such moments. In this case, a son who lived out of town and a daughter who lived nearby had different views on how to proceed. "Ethical dilemmas pit the good guys against the good guys," an experienced hospice nurse once taught the class. When struggles surface about what to do next, how to begin to solve a seemingly unsolvable ethical dilemma, it is usually safe, until proved otherwise, to assume that everyone's intentions are good.

Finally we asked not only, "What's this like for the patient and the patient's family," but also, "What's this like for the physician, the social worker, the nurse, the chaplain, and all others who participate in the patient's care? What can we learn from each other?" We learned that the professionals shared insights about care, validated and critiqued each others' conclusions, experienced loss, and supported each other.

GENUINE COLLABORATION

Care often involves a complex collaboration among many professionals. When we collaborate—*genuinely* collaborate—we enhance our ability to serve our patients, streamline care, and generate ongoing opportunities to learn and enhance trust.[5] Absence of collaboration can adversely influence outcome or delay recovery as much as incorrect diagnosis or inappropriate treatment can.

We can learn a great deal from the following two contrasting stories, chosen because they involve collaboration among various health professionals rather than solely among physicians.

Case 1: A Story with No Collaboration

A 72-year-old widow had diabetes, hypertension, and a seizure disorder for several years. On a day when her blood sugar concentration was very high, she fainted. Her physician concluded that neither her previously diagnosed seizure disorder and hypertension nor the drugs she was taking caused the collapse. He increased the dose of her diabetes pills, and she had no recurrence.

Though she had had diabetes for many years, she had no obvious complications of it. Her vision, kidney function, and circulation were good. She was not depressed, and her memory was sound. She had moved to an apartment after her husband's death several years previously, lived alone in a small apartment, spent time with friends, and occupied herself with various activities outside her home. Her children lived nearby and looked in on her frequently.

Her blood sugar concentration remained elevated, though she did not feel ill. Nevertheless, her physician decided that her diabetes was inadequately controlled on oral medicine and that she needed to take insulin injections. He felt that she had neither the dexterity nor the intellectual capacity to administer her own injections and recommended that she move to a nursing home. The visiting nurse endorsed that view and, when the patient declined, threatened to "report her to the county adult protection agency." When her daughter made an initial inquiry at nursing home about fees, she was told that they "would have to pay $3,000 up front."

Given the choice between "better control of her diabetes" in a nursing home and independent living, the patient chose to remain at home. Dissatisfied with her physician, her nurse, and "the system," she sought an opinion from another doctor.

Her physician had identified all her medical problems and he had care-fully addressed the potential causes of her episode of collapse. The nurse had visited her periodically to assess the efficacy of her treatment. The nursing home social worker had provided information to the patient and her daughter when they inquired about the process of nursing home admis-sion. But when each of them was called upon to help the patient and her family make a complex decision about her care and living arrangements, they failed. They neither worked together nor talked it over with each other. They failed to involve the patient and her family in examining the alternatives. They provided information without context. They assessed the medical and technical issues but neglected the patient's resources, val-ues, and preference for independent living. She dismissed them all!

Case 2: A Story with Genuine Collaboration

A 73-year-old man with long-standing diabetes was referred to the social worker by his home care nurse. He had become almost completely blind in the pre-vious eight months, had poor leg circulation, a foot ulcer, hypertension, partial pa-ralysis from a stroke, and was depressed. When the nurse became concerned about his ability to manage independently at home, she discussed his problems with the social worker and arranged a joint meeting with the patient, the nurse, the social worker, and the patient's son and daughter-in-law, also a nurse.

During this meeting, they discussed home care options and addressed his ongo-ing needs. All agreed to avoid the patient's moving from home for as long as possi-ble, and they explored ways to accomplish this goal: a live-in companion who would do household tasks in exchange for room and board, a homemaker to assist in daytime needs when the person sharing the home was away, and a volunteer vis-itor through the neighborhood "Block Nurse" program. They agreed on referrals to the Society for the Blind for assistance in training for use of his kitchen, to a physi-cal therapist to give home instruction on the use of a lightweight walker, to an oc-cupational therapist who arranged for bathroom safety apparatus, and to a psychologist to help him deal with his depression.

With the concurrence of this physician, all of these suggestions were imple-mented. With each referral to and conversation with another agency or resource, the social worker provided context to each new participant in the patient's care: not only the list of his medical problems but also his story and special needs. Throughout his care, the social worker and the nurse provided emotional support to the patient and his family and coordinated all the services provided. Once, when he became weak and unsteady, the nurse questioned whether his blood pres-sure medicine was the cause and she called his physician, who decreased the dose; the patient's symptoms improved.

From the beginning, the patient and his family were involved in defining the issues, exploring solutions, and making decisions. The patient's values were immediately identified and integrated into his plan of care. All of the involved professionals knew the patient's whole story, not simply that of his illness. There was ease of communication among the professionals. By sharing information, they facilitated important technical decisions—the decision about his blood pressure medication, for instance.

Each of these two stories asked the questions, "What's best for the patient?" and "Where should the patient live?" But the processes differed. One worked, the other did not, and the outcomes were different also. What do we learn from these stories? What is the difference in the approaches? And what can we learn about *genuine collaboration?*

In genuine collaboration, all those who need to be involved are consulted. Though the means of inquiry, data gathering, and testing may differ among the professions, each operates from the same story about the patient and has similar goals. The goals are negotiable; where conflict exists between professionals or between a professional and the patient, those conflicts are recognized and clarified, for they often represent disparate or incomplete versions of the same story.

In genuine collaboration, the patient and the family—sometimes the forgotten partners in collaboration—take part in the decisions. Ultimately, unless the patient is incompetent, she has the final approval. The patient and family may have insights about the cause and unique behavior of the illness, prior treatment attempts, what helped, what did not, and what made things worse. These observations help to streamline care and prevent catastrophe.

In genuine collaboration, there are ongoing critical review and oversight. As the story evolves, the character of the illness and the needs and the resources may change, and so the goals may need to be altered. In any complex system of care, the process may falter, but each participant knows that it can be fixed by talking it over. Genuine collaboration allows everyone the opportunity to validate their information and their approach to problems, and to alter the plan of care as often as necessary.

In genuine collaboration, one person is in charge. Otherwise, no one is in charge, or someone takes charge who may be the inappropriate person, or the patient and the family have to take charge by default, even though they may prefer not to. Such occurrences increase the risk for failure.

In genuine collaboration, no artificial boundaries exist between the professions; each has equal worth. The physician recognizes that some problems require neither tests nor physical remedies but rather attention to psychological or social issues. Others recognize the need for a physician's expertise. The professionals involved are at ease speaking with each other, sharing insights about the patient's care, and drawing from each others' expertise. They are part of an alliance, with each other and with the patient and his family. It is a comfortable alliance built on mutual trust. Often enough, the medical issues are but a few of the overall issues.

Genuine collaboration is liberating. From time to time, each professional is faced with tasks that exceed her skills. Tackling them alone is inefficient and unsatisfying. Calling upon others speeds up the process and allows each to concentrate on what she does best.

Genuine collaboration takes time. Attending to the whole story of the patient's illness and the psychological and social context in which it occurs, reflecting on the meaning of the information, identifying, clarifying, and validating the issues among all the participants, evolving a strategy for care and altering it when appropriate take time. But in the end, it is far more efficient than *not* collaborating, because all of the collaborating partners do their jobs with special skill.

Genuine collaboration allows the patient to develop trust in the system. Trust is reciprocal. When we trust and respect patients for their observations and personal values, they can trust those upon whose expertise they rely.

Genuine collaboration gives everyone an ongoing opportunity to learn. From other professionals, we learn better ways to explore the patient's story, to identify the issues, and to enlarge our knowledge of resources. We learn what works and what does not. By sharing our observations and inferences with others, we correct each others' misperceptions.

We also learn from our patients. This patient taught me a valuable lesson.

After her fifth hospitalization for congestive heart failure, each of which required the help of a consulting cardiologist and the use of a complex combination of medicines and electrical cardioversion, an 80-year-old patient thanked me with the statement of praise: "You've done it again!" I protested, "But Miss Dalton, it wasn't me; it was the cardiologist."[6] With a smile she replied, "Know your resources."

"Know your resources" is a multidimensional lesson. We must recognize that the patient, the family, and the community can be prime resources. We must know when the needs exceed our own skills and resources, when collaboration is necessary, and where to turn. We must know not only the institutional resources, but the people within them and how they work. Can we trust their perceptions and assessments? Are they thoughtful, or do they jump to conclusions? Are they consistent in their approaches? Do they ask, "What can I learn from this patient and from others with whom I work?" Do they *genuinely* collaborate? Such collaborative relationships are worth fostering. We must know what questions to ask and be able to formulate the questions clearly, and the person on either end of the consultation must know when to expand the inquiry.

"Know your resources" means "know your limitations"; but it also means "appreciate yourself as a resource." Often we can do more than we realize, just by thinking it over. Then we become our own consultant.

Chapter 13

Rituals

"The practice of medicine is full of rituals."

As part of everyday life, rituals help. Repetitive and reproducible, they provide pathways for action, especially when we do not quite know what to do. We turn to established rituals in dealing with moments in the cycle of life—death, marriage, and other passages, for those rituals are tested and refined by use. Religious liturgy is, of course, a ritual; it provides a set of prayers, in a certain order, with prescribed responses, and all of these elements help both the novice and the experienced.

The practice of medicine is full of rituals that help both the novice and the experienced physician. The method of taking the medical history is a ritual. It has an order and a way of expanding the questioning, is reproducible from patient to patient, is accepted by both the physician and the patient, and it works. If one is a novice, the history-taking "ritual" provides the structure for collecting and handling information. An experienced physician, even a tired one, can fall back on this ritual to guide the transaction.

The questions we ask and the problem-oriented system are among the rituals of diagnosis. Anticipating what can go wrong and instructing the patient, "Call me if you're not better by tomorrow" are treatment rituals. Some physicians, when they take their leave of patients, automatically, ritualistically, say, "I hope you feel better," a valediction not unlike a blessing.

There are rituals by which physicians communicate with one another: presenting the history, findings on patients' physical examinations, and test results, all leading to a diagnosis. As we listen and identify unanswered questions and issues, we can quickly focus.

But rituals sometimes can get in the way of original thinking. If, as physicians, we routinely obtain an electrocardiogram to rule out a heart problem and the test is normal, we may stop the diagnostic pursuit prematurely and squander the opportunity to enter into a productive conversation with the patient and explore the other possible causes of chest pain, including the human side. Bursztajn and his colleagues reflect: "Technical procedures, valuable as they are when there is a rational basis for using them, are invoked mindlessly and automatically, as rituals to reassure anxious physicians. Precise laboratory measurement is accepted as a substitute for a complex, elusive reality that may be understood only with patience and sensitivity."[1]

Rituals do not replace thoughtful discourse. Asking the patient to sign a permit for an operation does not substitute for talking about her fears. Speaking with a family about a "do not resuscitate" direction for their comatose parent does not substitute for a long talk about the meaning of their impending loss.

Certain rituals are missing in most medical settings. When someone dies in the hospital or nursing home after a long illness, a physician or nurse "pronounces the person dead," invasive tubes are removed, and the patient's body is moved to the institutional morgue to await transport to a funeral home. To address the loss for staff who have cared for the patient, an additional ritual can provide meaning to the entire experience and allow them to move on. Together they could recite a brief liturgy—no need to call it a "prayer"—acknowledging the worth of the deceased, the privilege of caring for him, and their own loss.

After a patient dies, another ritual helps to complete the chapter of care. When writing the survivors to express sympathy, we also declare what the relationship meant to us. In our letter, we may comment on some of the patient's special qualities. We may write, "You did all you possibly could. I hope that the many good memories you have of him will ease your grief in the months to come. Please let me know if I can help." We acknowledge the family's relationship to the patient and the magnitude of their loss. We offer our availability, for their drama is not yet over. Such letters can help to prevent their appropriate grief from turning into prolonged depression.

Coupled with the best rituals from medicine are the personal rituals of the patient and those derived from the patient's family, ethnic, and religious background. As potential resources, they all help.

Chapter 14

Language and Communication

"How do I know what I have said until I know what you have heard?"

Once, after being introduced to an audience of nurses to whom I spoke about the medical needs of recent Russian Jewish immigrants, I began my talk in Yiddish. "Don't panic," I said, switching to English after a few sentences and letting them in on my prank, "but think of what it would be like if you didn't understand what was going on in your new country. Think also what you would feel like if you didn't understand what your doctor was saying to you about a matter of great importance." The body of my talk dealt with the immigrant's adjustment to life in the United States and to the American system of medical care, but I used it as a metaphor. Any barrier to understanding gets in the way of productive discourse. Complete understanding and "speaking the same language" facilitate important decisions and genuine collaboration. There is no comparison between a conversation between a patient and physician allied with each other and one that is confrontational, patronizing, or full of jargon.

There are many superb transactions by which physicians communicate facts, opinions, consistency, reliability, accessibility, and commitment:

- "I can imagine what this must be like for you."
- "We'll do all we can to make this surgery turn out well."

- "Come down to the office this morning." (Not, "I'll see if I can fit you in.")
- "I don't know the answer, but I do know that it's nothing to be concerned about."
- "I don't know the answer, but I'll find out and call you in the next two days."
- "Here is what I think is wrong. . . ."

But there are barriers to communication. The concept of "language barrier" applies not only to the difference between the native language of the doctor and the patient but even between them when they share a language.

By reading between the lines, we enhance our understanding of what the patient means:

- When the husband of a deceased patient said to the physician, "You didn't do enough," he really was saying, "I wonder if *I* didn't do enough." The physician recognized this and used the criticism as an opportunity to address the husband's guilt and to reassure him that he had done all he possibly could.
- When, many years after the death of her retarded son, his mother declared that "I should have done more to prevent his death," the physician saw the opportunity to explore the meaning of her statement and gain further insight into her long-standing depression.
- The unexpected question from an 80-year-old patient, "What's my cholesterol?" was her way of asking, "How much longer do I have? How's my heart?"
- When a patient with widespread cancer asked, "How long do I have to live?" the physician realized she was not looking for a numerical answer. Rather she saw the opportunity to discuss the patient's goals and values and to address other unasked but implied questions: "Will I have uncontrollable pain? What will the remaining time be like?"

Unless the physician and the patient have a common understanding of the illness, they will have difficulty working together:

- A 75-year-old patient refused to restart insulin despite a very high blood sugar concentration, because she felt her sugar was "not that high," and she had also concluded that *only* those people who took insulin later lost their vision or needed leg amputations.
- A 50-year-old woman refused to take a cholesterol-lowering medicine because she feared its side-effects.
- A patient delayed prostate surgery for two years of unnecessary discomfort because his first doctor did a poor job of presenting his proposal. "If my original urologist had talked to me the way this last one did, I would have had surgery two years ago. He showed me the x-rays, he explained, he took the time."

When the patient becomes silent, the physician often has to subdue the urge to fill the silence quickly with a comment, an assurance, or another question. But patients pause for various reasons: to deal with painful thoughts, to stifle tears or other signs of emotions, or to plan what they are going to say next. Often what a patient says immediately after a period of silence has great significance, and to interrupt a silence is as inappropriate as interrupting a narration. Silence may provide an added dimension to what has been said. "In her silence," one student observed, "you felt that it was even more painful [than she described it]." Silence may allow both the patient and the physician time to reflect on what has been said—and left unsaid. There is *metaphoric* silence also, the absence of timely information, the absence of appropriately shared feelings. Some things are better said than left alone.

Words can harm. The physician may describe a patient as "manipulative," "hysterical," "noncompliant," or "a hypochondriac" and a family as "dysfunctional." Used carelessly and pejoratively, they cloud precise thinking. A single word cannot completely define patients or their families, until we know more about their stories, motivations, points of view, reasons for behavior, and values.

Physicians especially need to choose words carefully. Some years ago, my patient went to a nearby medical center for a second opinion about what he thought were episodes of hypoglycemia. After having been interviewed by the resident-in-training and going through several days of tests, he saw the senior physician. When he finished retelling his story at this long-anticipated meeting, the doctor said, "Mr. R, I have never heard a story like yours before." What the doctor meant was, "You don't have hypoglycemia. Your story doesn't sound like it," but any reasonable patient could have thought, "If you've never heard a story like this before, I think I'd like to see someone who *has*. That's why I'm here, at great inconvenience and expense." What physicians say may mean something entirely different than intended to the listener, because it is unclear, because the listener is tense, or because the listener does not understand the physician's language, even though they are both speaking English. As one student put it, "How do I know what I have said until I know what you have heard?"

Here are some other examples of what is said and what is heard:

- When a physician told a 27-year-old man, a heavy drinker, that "your liver tests are abnormal," the patient concluded that he had irreversible and fatal liver disease. The physician needed to explain that the abnormalities were reversible, and he needed to say it more than once.

- When the physician told a patient, "You have arthritis," she heard, "I'm falling apart. I'm going to become disabled with a crippling disease." She needed a detailed explanation that the "arthritis" to which he referred was the type that would not become disabling.

- When a patient asked the cardiologist, "Will the Lanoxin [that he was taking for a disorder of his heart rhythm] hurt my heart?" she replied, "It's hardly therapeutic." What she meant was, "It's not at a dangerous level." The patient's interpretation: "If it's not therapeutic, then why am I taking it?"

- "You have hypertension" was a statement of trivial importance to the physician, because high blood pressure is so common. To one patient, it meant imminent stroke, a lifetime of medicine with adverse effects, and the transition from perfect health to a flawed body.

- The urologist told a patient with prostate cancer, previously treated with surgery, that his prostate-specific antigen (PSA) blood test level, used to follow the progress of the disease, had increased slightly and should be repeated in six months rather than a year. The physician was only expressing the need for more diligent surveillance. The effect on the patient was profound: Concerned that his tumor was progressing, he became anxious and depressed.

"Lack of clarity equals bad news," a friend observed after he had listened to a cardiologist present a jargon-filled description of his father's coronary angiogram. Physicians who stumble with complex explanations are often struggling with their own difficulty in delivering bad news. Even if they are not, it is too easy for patients to misinterpret and infer the worst. A patient once told me, "What the doctor tells me has a profound effect on my mind."

Even the way we address patients carries weight. Greeting an adult patient for the first time with "Hi, Harry" initiates a different quality of transaction than "How do you do, Mr. Swenson." The first greeting lacks the respect and deference due any person. Many will prefer to be addressed more informally by their first name, but it is their call, not the physician's.

Any patient's question becomes an opportunity to engage in discussion and explore issues. Good physicians read between the lines and ask themselves, "What does my patient's question mean?" To the patient, they say, "I want to be certain I understand. Tell me what you mean when you say. . . ." Patients survive bad language and communication, but why cause additional pain? Reflecting on his heart attack, Arthur Frank wrote: "The more extreme the situation, the more time and help I need to say anything. . . . You cannot be told that you have had a heart attack without having a great deal to express and needing to express it. The problem is finding someone who will help you work out the terms of that expression."[1]

Sometimes the disparity in understanding is not so obvious, often signaled by an inappropriately angry response to advice. This conversation—between a physician and the son of an elderly nursing home patient after his mother had become more confused—illustrates:

Physician: There's a possibility that she may have fallen, struck her head, and developed a subdural hematoma, a blood clot pressing on her brain.

Son: I don't think she has a blood clot.

Physician: That's a decision for *me*.

The son took offense. What he meant was, "I want to keep my prerogatives, since I know my mother best of all." What the physician meant was, "You need not have the burden of deciding if she has a blood clot; that's what you have a doctor for." The physician was wise enough to recognize this discrepancy in interpretation immediately, and they were able to come to an accommodation: Even if there was a strong likelihood for the hematoma, they decided together, nothing would be done therapeutically, and so no further tests would be done. When patients or families become angry, physicians need to ask, "What does my patient's anger mean?" Patients may be angry for various reasons. Misunderstanding is at the top of the list, which includes depression, a prior unpleasant transaction with a physician, frustration with the "system," frustration with an illness that is not going well, and unrevealed psychological issues.

WHAT DO WE LEARN?

Here are some lessons I have learned over the years about language and communication.

Sit. Do not minimize the importance of body language. Sitting when one talks with a patient is an important gesture. No matter if the conversation is less than a minute, patients see this as a commitment to them and them alone, a statement that "you are all I have on my mind now." Less than a minute sitting seems like five minutes standing. Five minutes standing seems as if "the doctor's got one foot out the door."

Talk with patients as equals. Do not talk down. Do not shout. Here is one of my favorite stories. Early in my career, I assumed that all old people were hearing impaired, and so I introduced myself to an 89-year-old woman by shouting, "I'm Dr. Savett!" She responded in kind, "Good for you!"

Set the context. In order to explain things to patients, provide a context and start where the patient is. I often begin with a general statement such as "All in all, I think your health is good." Then I continue with the details of the diagnosis and other issues of concern. When necessary, I enlarge the context. For example, each time she came to the office, a 45-year-old attorney dwelled on her obesity, her unresponsiveness to diet, and her poor image of herself. We enlarged the context by talking about her successful roles as mother, wife, and competent legal advocate.

Make no assumptions about the patient's level of knowledge. Even if the patient is a professional colleague, state the assumptions, clarify them if necessary, be certain of agreement, and try to understand all the participants in the drama. Ask, "What have you been told so far?"

Explore the patient's beliefs and values. My new patient, a 95-year-old Orthodox Jew, had a seizure just before he was brought to the hospital. Though the emergency had passed, he was still unconscious, and I was concerned that we might be faced with more acute problems and have to make urgent judgments about treatment and especially about resuscitation. I spoke with his daughter about "comfort, pain, and dignity" and suggested hospitalization and forgoing resuscitation. She insisted that we "do everything" including resuscitation. In their tradition, she taught me, the soul is that which should be preserved, and the body, the container of the soul, should therefore be preserved as long as possible, for in those additional moments, important insights may occur and relationships may be healed.

That discussion reinforced lessons about dealing with *all* patients, the need to inquire about beliefs and values and be aware that words mean different things to different people. To me, the "dignity" of hospitalization that I proposed meant a comforting bedside scene; to the family, it meant the intrusion of repeated trips to the hospital to visit, a far less attractive choice than nursing him at home with family always present. To me, "pain" meant the pain of resuscitation; to them, it meant the pain of premature loss.

In helping patients to make a difficult decision, I often ask them to consider two questions: "Is it, the treatment, worth it?" and "Am I, the patient, worth it?" If both of your answers to those questions are "yes," I tell them, then the other decisions will flow from that. And if both answers are not "yes," we need to explore their values.

Recognize that a long conversation is often better than a short one. In the midst of a patient's long hospitalization for liver disease, a nonmalignant ovarian tumor, and many surgical complications, I talked for an hour with her and her husband. During this time, I reviewed the entire hospitalization, how we had gotten to where we were (she was still seriously ill), inquired about prior crises they had faced and their strengths during those times, expressed hope for a quick recovery, assured them of my commitment to do all I could, and recognized the uncertainties. We could not have addressed all these issues in a brief time, nor could a few short conversations have explored them in depth.

Recognize that a confrontation is often an indication for a longer conversation. A face-to-face conversation is better than a phone call. When the physician sees a patient rather than simply talking on the phone, the transaction carries more weight. The patient perceives: She cares enough to see me, to take the time, and to look me over. Not only does the patient hear the physician's voice, but he sees her face and body language, all of which enhance the value of her decisions and instructions.

Authorize the patient to speak freely. "I want you to know that there is nothing we can't talk about. And if you don't understand what I have said or if you disagree, you should let me know." Acknowledge that "you wouldn't be human if you weren't apprehensive." Ask, "What about this surgery frightens you the most?"

Negotiate. I propose a theory of the illness or a remedy, and then the patient and I refine it. I ask, "Does this sound reasonable to you?" and allow the conversation to evolve. I never forget that patients are expert and have first-hand knowledge about their symptoms, reaction to certain drugs, and the impact of life's events on their health. A 40-year-old bachelor described chest pain that I thought was similar to pain he had had for over twenty years. He was out of work, and he was concerned that he had heart trouble. After carefully listening to him and examining him, I said, "I think your pain is likely not related to your heart, especially in view of what's going on in your life." His response was, "But this pain is different—the location is different." As we talked further, it became clear to me that this pain required further investigation, including evaluation for heart disease. That is why I reason out loud, in order that together we can decide if the decisions are appropriate.

Tell stories. To get information or to make a point, I tell a story that may have some parallel to the dilemma. To a man whose wife had just died, I said, "One of my patients, a man your age, felt as if he was losing his mind when his wife died. What does your wife's death mean to you?" The story authorized him to talk about his feelings, something he was not used to doing. To the son who is struggling with a decision to forgo resuscitation on his terminally ill father, I told the story of a similar moment in author Philip Roth's life, when he whispered to his unconscious father, dying from a brain tumor, "Dad, I'm going to have to let you go."[2]

Acknowledge reality. "You'll be OK" may be an appropriate assessment, but it is inadequate in some situations. To the patient who was recovering from a heart attack and had real fears about the future, I said, "I know that what will reassure you the most is first getting two weeks and then two months of good health behind you."

Recognize that not all questions have answers. Acknowledge uncertainty, but set time limits. A 50-year-old bus driver had pain in his abdomen for two months. His story suggested duodenal ulcer, and I treated him with antiulcer medication. "Let's give it a try for two weeks. If it's not better, then we need to do some more tests." Most people can handle the uncertainty.

Deliver difficult news face to face and with compassion. "You're carrying a pregnancy that has a birth defect incompatible with life," a patient's obstetrician told her. Just like that. She fired the obstetrician. Allow patients to absorb the bad news, reflect, and then talk about their feelings. Ask, "What's this like for you?"

Write letters of condolence. Writing condolence letters is a ritual I described in the last chapter. I often write to the nurses who have been so closely involved in the patient's care, for I recognize their loss also.

TEACHING ABOUT LANGUAGE AND COMMUNICATION

Developing a warm communication style takes practice. Watching videotapes of interviews (including our own), role playing, and then critiquing the exercise work in a trusting environment. When what we say to a patient is misunderstood, the critical physician will ask, "Why didn't this work? How can I say it better? What can I learn so that next time I'll do it better?"

To teach undergraduates and pediatric residents about language and communication, I use a story about a 21-month-old boy who had been in good health until his father left home.[3] When his mother began abusing alcohol and neglecting him, he developed recurring middle ear infections and lost weight. His hometown physician sent him to the infectious diseases clinic at the nearby medical center. After a few appointments, he was hospitalized there for "failure to thrive, feeding problems, developmental delay, and recurrent otitis media (middle ear infections)." An extensive evaluation with multiple tests followed. Each time he ran a fever, he had more tests; none was conclusive. The intern assigned to his case recognized that he was continuing to decline and that there might be another approach to his care. Especially since the tests were not helpful, there seemed to be no point in repeating them each time the child had a fever, and so each episode of fever was treated with antibiotics without further investigation. In addition, the intern, with the help of a compassionate volunteer, concentrated on his feeding and providing a safe, consistent environment. The child rallied. "[The intern] continued to treat [the toddler] as his personal responsibility and to act as his physician [and] 'advocate.' "

I ask each student to assume that he or she is the toddler's physician, who wishes to share the uncertainties of the diagnosis and treatment with his mother in a way that is realistic yet does not promote panic. "What else do you want this conversation to accomplish?" I ask them. "What would you say?"

Here is what one group of students wanted this conversation to accomplish. They wanted to establish their credentials, credibility, and reliability; get more information about the child; find out what is going on in the mother's life and what this experience is like for her; discover her understanding of the illness; review all the important information with the mother; talk about the diagnosis, treatment, prognosis, and uncertainties; ask about her wishes for her child; address the necessity for her to be more responsible; begin to explore referral to a social worker and child care classes; reinforce good behavior; establish a trusting alliance; and assure the mother that she does not have to handle this situation alone and will not be abandoned.

During the exercise, a number of things occurred. Some who played the doctor role presented all of this material in a thoughtful, compassionate, and understandable way. Others talked endlessly, without stopping to allow the mother to ask questions. They spoke in a patronizing tone and used medical jargon. ("The blood tests have not shown any definable illness. His white count is elevated. He may have an immunologic disease.") Ultimately they all recognized that they should "speak her language," be certain that both she and the physician were using the same information, make no assumptions without validating them with her, say the important things more than once, and do it all in a way that was respectful, reassuring, and not officious. Of course, I ask the students, "What did you learn? In what way can the lessons from this story and these exercises influence your approach to learning and to patient care?"

When physicians share responsibilities for care with colleagues, they must speak a language that each understands. In conversations with physicians, patients deserve no less. A caption in the Minnesota Historical Society exhibit on "Minnesota Communities" concluded, "When you find someone who 'speaks your language,' you experience an immediate and lasting bond."[4]

Chapter 15

===

What Can Go Wrong

"A succession of errors made and learned from."
—Henry Louis Gates, Jr.

If only the practice of medicine were as simple as, "When illness A is treated with treatment B, everything turns out OK." But even with the best of intentions, faulty judgments and hubris, unquestioning pride in one's own opinion, may derail appropriate action, harm the patient, and teach the wrong lessons. Part of being a good doctor is recognizing these potential pitfalls and learning from our own mistakes.

TREATMENT-INDUCED ILLNESS

Treatment with both prescribed and "over-the-counter" drugs, surgery, and other procedures may make patients and their illnesses worse.[1] Even simple maneuvers carry risks; prolonged bed rest predisposes to pneumonia, phlebitis (blood clots), and bedsores. Treatment-induced illness is so common that the physician should consider it whenever a patient presents a new problem. Delay in the diagnosis of treatment-induced illness may prolong an illness, adversely affect the outcome, lead to unnecessary and costly evaluation, prolong an inappropriate treatment, and place the patient in future jeopardy from the unrecognized offender. These two cases illustrate.

Case 1

An 81-year-old woman, a nursing home resident, was hospitalized after a day of fever and abdominal pain. She was confused on admission, and physical and x-ray examinations of the chest showed evidence of pneumonia. Because of the confusion and fever, she had a lumbar puncture (a spinal tap); the results were normal. She had been taking a number of medicines: a mild sedative, calcium and vitamin D for osteoporosis, and twelve adult aspirin a day for aching joints. Blood calcium level was normal, but the salicylate level, an index of aspirin toxicity, was markedly elevated. The physician prescribed penicillin for the pneumonia, discontinued the aspirin, and began treatment for salicylate intoxication. Within three days, her pneumonia and mental status improved.

In this case, the patient was seriously ill with pneumonia and unexplained abdominal pain. The physician could have concluded that her confusion was a manifestation of her other serious problems or the disorientation often observed in elderly persons suddenly moved to a strange setting. By reviewing her drug history, her physician recognized and addressed each treatable drug-induced cause of the confusion: too much sedation, an increased concentration of calcium, and chronic salicylate intoxication from aspirin.

Case 2

When his employer became concerned about his reliability and erratic behavior, a 35-year-old engineer saw a new physician. Previously an excellent worker, in the last few months, he could no longer concentrate and had lost interest in his job. For sixteen years, he had taken insulin for diabetes. Because of this recent change in his mental status, the physician hospitalized him. On the first day, he reduced his insulin dose by 25 percent, and even then an insulin reaction occurred. By the time of discharge, the patient was receiving an even smaller dose and was able to concentrate, and he was soon "back to his old self."

Had his erratic behavior been explained as a primary psychiatric disorder, his problem would not have been solved. Recurring hypoglycemic reactions from too much insulin were responsible.

There are many reasons for failure or delay in the diagnosis of treatment-induced illness. The physician may not even consider this possibility. More than one physician may be prescribing and treating a patient. The physician may be unaware of all the potential side effects of the drugs and treatments the patient is using. The combination of problems may be so complex that other illnesses overshadow the drug-related aspect. The new problem may be considered a sign or symptom of an ongoing previously identified problem and therefore ignored. The interval between the initial prescription of the drug and the onset of the drug-induced illness may be of sufficient length that the physician fails to connect the two events. The treatment-induced illness may not be sufficiently dramatic to be brought to the physician's attention. It is hard for the patient to ignore a rash that itches and might be caused by penicillin; it is easier to overlook mild depression caused by a blood pressure medicine.

No physician can know every adverse effect of every drug and treatment, and so we must have a strategy for recognizing treatment-induced illness. The important steps are (1) Identify and name the problem; for example, "confusion" or "fever" or "change in mental status." (2) Ask, "Why now? Is there some precipitating cause for the new problem?" (3) Ask, "Is the new problem caused by the treatment of an existing problem?" Involve patients in their own care by encouraging them to report any new symptoms or deterioration in their feeling of well-being. And, even though it is not literally true, always use this rule of thumb: Any drug can cause any side effect.

PREJUDICE

Generalizations help us make decisions. Unless we can provide some classification and grouping to persons, patients, illnesses, and symptoms, we will be forced to address each new problem as a completely new task. We will be unable to call on experience. When physicians define a patient too narrowly, they forgo creative ways of looking at their problems; prejudice gets in the way of diagnosis and treatment. Prejudice means "an adverse judgment or opinion formed beforehand or without knowledge or examination of the facts; a preconceived preference or idea."[2]

I teach about prejudice by drawing on students' own experiences. At their age, they have already been discriminated against because they are not Caucasian, not Protestant, gay or lesbian, or young or have diabetes. They have even been discriminated against because they are students! The list is endless. This story, told by an older student, is an example.

Case 3

Several years ago, my partner and I went on a skiing vacation in Colorado. When we left, [he] had a cold and a deep chest cough. After arriving, we started skiing, and while riding the gondola to the top of the mountain, [he] complained of shortness of breath, fatigue, and a general feeling of malaise. Throughout the afternoon, he became more tired. . . . We quit skiing early that day. . . . By the time he went to bed, he was coughing heavily and complained again about being light-headed.

[The next] morning, he was coughing up blood and said he had not slept at all during the night. . . . [As the day progressed, he became] very lethargic and continued to cough up blood. I insisted that we go to the hospital to have him checked out. . . . I was aware that [he] had almost died when he was very young from pneumonia. . . .

The doctor came out with an x-ray, . . . pointed to several small white spots on the x-ray, and told [us] that they looked like *Pneumocystis* pneumonia (a serious infection often associated with AIDS). Until further tests were conducted, however, he could not be sure. He said he had seen many cases of *Pneumocystis* in gay men when he worked at a hospital that had an AIDS clinic. . . . [He] asked if [we] had ever had an HIV test. I told him we both had been tested and the results were negative. He said he would . . . start treating him with a course of drugs used to treat HIV-related *Pneumocystis*. Another test would also be done to confirm his HIV status. . . . It was Friday afternoon, and a million things were going through our heads. Some of them were thoughts we shared. The others were our personal fears, anger, and anxiety about how we were going to deal with the situation. . . .

[After three days of treatment, another doctor] introduced himself as the staff internist and told us that . . . the HIV results were negative and that in his opinion, [my partner] had been suffering from a severe case of high-altitude sickness that was complicated by his chest cold. The spots on the lungs appeared to be from the pneumonia he had when he was a child. His best advice was to get to a lower altitude as soon as possible. He apologized for the misdiagnosis by the other doctor and tried to explain how it happened. Four hours later, and 9,000 feet lower, [my partner's] color returned, his breathing became easier, and his mood was vastly improved.

Our experience turned out to have a happy ending. However, after going through the experience, I could not help but empathize with the thousands of people who never get that second chance to have an AIDS diagnosis reversed and how they must feel when confronted with the news. I also realized the importance of questioning medical professionals about a diagnosis and the importance of being actively involved in the decisions that are made. Most importantly, I learned that doctors make mistakes just like anyone else, and that patients' and their families' rights and feelings must always be respected.

The first doctor's reasoning probably went like this: *Seriously ill gay man with respiratory symptoms and abnormal chest x-ray* equals *AIDS-related pneumonia.* All of this could have been avoided had he reflected, "Could the abnormal chest x-ray be related to any other problems, such as his pneumonia when younger? What else could this be?" Instead, his premature conclusion delayed the correct diagnosis and treatment and devastated the patient and his partner.

Prejudice undermines each step of the "five-step paradigm" (chapter 1). It interferes with obtaining the whole *story*, and so it weakens the accuracy of the derived *history*. It intrudes on the accurate definition of the *issues*, including diagnosis and treatment. It subverts the *doctor-patient relationship*. Prejudice *teaches the wrong lessons*. When they are perpetuated and integrated into the physician's way of practice, they can cause mayhem.

Here are some other examples of prejudice:

- Because a patient speaks no English, she is treated as someone who "does not understand," of limited intellectual capacity. Non-English-speaking patients have the same illnesses, vulnerabilities, and intelligence as English speakers.
- The characterization, "All [insert any immigrant group name] are difficult to deal with" denies the patient *and* the physician the opportunity to ask, "What's this all about?" In the former Soviet Union, for example, patients had to challenge the system aggressively in order to get attention, and so why would they think differently about the system in the United States before they learned otherwise?
- "He's depressed because he was a prisoner in a concentration camp." Never mind looking into other aspects of his life—that he has lost his job, that his wife is unfaithful, that he is unable to pay his bills. But not every Holocaust survivor is depressed. Explaining away the depression denies the physician and the patient the benefit of examining all the factors we would ordinarily examine in a depressed person, starting with the losses: loss of family, home, and country.
- "She's rebellious because she has diabetes." This invalid inference squanders the opportunity to speak with the teenager about what is going on in her life and to find ways to help.

Patients have told me that they have been treated in a prejudiced way for other reasons: They are old, young, a woman, a widow, a blond, overweight, a person of color, tall, short, hard of hearing, on welfare, a "cancer patient," or a person with a foreign accent. Remember the physician recovering from coronary bypass surgery (chapter 1) to whom the nurse said, "I thought that because you are a doctor, you didn't need that kind of attention [to your feelings]." None of these characterizations is sufficient to define a person, any more than any illness name does. Terms like "diabetic" and "cancer patient" close down thoughtful consideration of who they are and what is wrong with them.

Patients have prejudices also. In the next chapter, I tell the story of a patient who dismissed a physician because she thought he dressed inappropriately. Patients may reject a physician because of youth, race, ethnic origin, gender, or other narrow reasons. But there is a difference between a patient's prejudices and those of a physician. While patients cannot always be expected to neutralize their prejudices in the encounter, physicians must do so, lest their judgment be impaired and actions affected. There is as much danger in jumping to conclusions about people as there is danger in jumping to conclusions about diagnosis and treatment. "Old" *may* mean "rigid and less inclined to change," but not necessarily. "Gay" *may* mean "at risk for developing AIDS," but not necessarily. "Having cancer" *may* mean "depressed," but not necessarily. A student observed, "When we are most resistant to maintaining an open mind, that is when we should be most critical of our thoughts and look for our prejudices."

ABUSE

Abuse[3] means "to hurt or injure by maltreatment."[4] We may abuse with our words, and even though we do so inadvertently rather than deliberately, the impact on the patient may be the same. I like the saying, "Never attribute to malice that which can adequately be explained by stupidity." Most physicians can recall moments when we or our colleagues have said the wrong thing or reacted strongly and inappropriately to a situation. The trick is to ask, "What can we learn from this transaction?" and then do it better the next time. Such lapses of professional behavior hurt the patient and the patient's family. Even when the outcome of an illness is good, the process of recovery can be emotionally painful. If physicians magnify the pain by their own behavior, then they have served their patient poorly. Early on we are taught, "First do no harm."

Here are some of the inadvertent ways we physicians abuse our patients and their families.

We are bigoted. We see patients not as individuals but as members of a group. We characterize them unfairly and inaccurately. We patronize them. We fail to recognize that each patient has many dimensions. The previous sections describe the dangers.

We do not understand. We do not comfort. When we do not start where the patient and the family are, we increase their pain. A surgeon spoke to the family of a 70-year-old woman after she had had a kidney removed because of cancer. The family needed to hear only that she had come through the surgery without difficulty, for they already knew that her illness had a poor prognosis. They also needed an expression of compassion. His first words to them were, "The horse is out of the barn! She has metastases."

We do not listen.

We provide information without context and prognosis, and so we may perpetuate uncertainty. A 35-year-old man developed ventricular extrasystoles, an irregular heartbeat, usually a benign condition causing "palpitations." After examining him, his physician ordered a succession of tests including a twenty-four-hour recording of his heartbeat, a cardiac ultrasound, and a cardiac stress test. After each test, he reported to the patient by telephone, "Your test was normal," but he never discussed the patient's fear of heart disease, nor did he say, "The rhythm abnormality is a common one. You need not be concerned." Lacking that reassurance, the patient sought further consultation.

We delegate inappropriately. We fail to recognize that the patient and the family need more than information. The message, "Your mammogram was abnormal," needs a conversation with the doctor. When we delegate the task of relaying a medical message to a person who is unable to provide more information, we increase the patient's discomfort. We build barriers instead of bridges by requiring patients to tell their stories to assistants, when they really need to talk with us.

We meet anger with anger. Instead, we should ask, "What does my patient's anger mean?" When we fail to interpret and address the anger and instead respond in kind, we increase the patient's discomfort.

We isolate. When we fail to explain, when we use jargon, when we fail to understand, when we take action without explaining why, when we assume patients know the answers when they do not, we increase their discomfort.

But none of these lapses is without remedy. As always, "a problem identified is a problem half solved." If, as physicians, we integrate awareness of these issues into our methods of practice and our professional curricula, continuing education courses, and ongoing evaluation of care, we go a long way toward providing comprehensive care. When we can recognize our deficiencies and learn from them, even our lapses become opportunities for professional growth.

MISTAKES

Most medical mistakes are made despite the best of intentions. We need only review the diary of a physician's day (chapters 8 and 22) to recognize how many decisions a physician makes each day. Despite the best of intentions, mistakes happen. Of retired Army General, and now Secretary of State, Colin Powell, Henry Louis Gates, Jr., wrote, "His narrative of those [army] years is a succession of errors made and learned from—mistakes transmuted into maxims. In time, he was happy enough to skip the mistakes part."[5]

I was unnerved by the first big mistake of which I was aware, when I was a medical resident. I recall it vividly. A 50-year-old man with chronic heart disease developed a disorder of his heart rhythm, which I thought was caused by digitalis, one of his medicines. I stopped the drug but forgot to re-start it a few days later at a lower dose. A week later, he developed serious heart failure and a cardiac arrest requiring emergency resuscitation. He sur-vived but died a week later. Although the underlying illness alone could have been responsible for the complications and death, I felt that what had happened was my fault; but for my error, none of this would have occurred. I felt alone and isolated. I spoke of my feelings with no one, for I felt that no one else had ever made a mistake of such magnitude and with such serious consequences. Had I discussed my feelings with a colleague, a teacher, or a peer, I would have learned more from the experience.

I know better now. The sheer number of decisions we make, alone or in conjunction with others, makes it impossible to have a perfect record. Of his own error, Dr. David Hilfiker, then practicing in a small town, wrote: "As a student, I was simply not aware that the sort of mistakes I would even-tually make in practice actually happened to competent physicians. . . . Physicians need permission to admit errors. They need permission to share them with their patients. The practice of medicine is difficult enough with-out having to bear the yoke of perfection."[6]

Now medical school curricula include lessons and discussions about mis-takes. There are errors of process: how physicians look at and manage a problem from beginning to end and how they communicate with a patient and family. Some errors reflect inadequate or incomplete knowledge: the failure to recognize an illness or the availability of a treatment option. Hilfiker describes mistakes resulting from not knowing enough, a lack of technical skill, simple carelessness, a failure of judgment, or what he calls "a failure of will . . . in which a doctor knows the right thing to do but doesn't do it because he is distracted, or pressured, or exhausted."[7] There are errors of omission and commission. Each of these kinds of mistakes has its own obvious remedy.

When we discover a mistake, we have a natural tendency to ask, "Whose fault is it? Was it the fault of the physician, the consultant, the nurse, the 'system'?" Or even, "Was it the patient's fault [for not informing me of a critical piece of information, for not following up, etc.]?" A better question is, "What happened?" Then we can take the next productive step by ask-ing, "What can we learn from this error?"

Mistakes may have little or no impact on patients; some are serious and contribute to a bad outcome, including death. They have impact on the physician also. A mistake may shake our confidence, and so we need strate-gies for dealing with mistakes.

The best strategy is to talk about mistakes. Medicine has several tradi-tions. One is "death and complications conferences," periodic reviews of unanticipated problems and poor outcomes. Another is "clinical pathological conferences," in which difficult diagnostic problems with ultimately known solutions are presented to a gathering of physicians and experts who analyze, step by step, the evolution of the case and the reasoning of the attending physicians. Talking about mistakes happens in an informal way also; physicians examine clinical mishaps, analyze what happened, and figure out ways to learn from them and do it better next time. Talking with a colleague about unsuccessful conversations with patients can provide the same benefit; we learn a better way to say what we have to say. We learn, so that we do not repeat our errors.

One of my students defined one characteristic of the physician as a professional when he wrote: "It is fair to criticize a doctor's inability to learn from a failure, but not to criticize the failure itself." Acknowledging mistakes and then learning from them are part of being a good physician and a real professional. The next chapter more completely addresses the question, "What is a professional?"

Chapter 16

The Physician as Professional

"Here is someone . . . who knows what she's doing."

My friend, a very good internist, had just started his practice in a small New England town and was making hospital rounds on his partner's patients one Saturday morning. In those days, the early 1970s, he was somewhat of a hippie and dressed the part—flannel shirt, sandals, beard, and ponytail. His first patient, an 80-year-old Yankee dowager, eyed him carefully—and promptly dismissed him. In a strong voice, she declared, "You won't do!" What she meant was, "I don't know you, but your appearance suggests to me that you're a bit odd, and what I need is a doctor, in the image of my current physician—a properly dressed man, a real professional." The packaging was wrong, and she would not look beyond that.

I tell my students this story in order to introduce the question, "What is a professional?" and to address the role of physician as professional. Is the physician merely a technician, educated in anatomy, histology, and the other basic sciences and skilled in diagnosis and treatment, or is there more? From whose standpoint should we address the question? The patient's? The physician's? The third parties'—hospitals, insurers, government, and related institutions? Or all of them?

A concerned family member gives advice to her relative with chest pain by saying, "When my husband had chest pain, his doctor gave him a stress test." The firefighter takes the blood pressure of someone who has a headache and says, "The blood pressure is normal." What does the physician do that these well-meaning people cannot? What makes the physician a professional? What qualities, if absent, are cause for change to another physician? Insights and answers to these come from listening to people in careers unrelated to medicine.

My long-time mechanic looks after my used Volvo. I am truly uninformed about the way my car works, and so when I take it in, I rely on him to provide answers. I listen to his explanation, for not only does he tell me what he proposes to do or what he has done, but he tells me why. More than a technician, he helps me understand what is wrong in language I understand. As my car has aged, he has told me what is worth fixing and what is not, and when it is time to give up and trade the car in. Even though he has a potential conflict of interest—he works fee-for-service and clearly makes a living from fixing cars—I trust that he will not take advantage of me. Our first encounter proved that. The rear of my car shook whenever I drove over twenty miles per hour. He discovered the cause, a tire that needed to be replaced, sent me to a tire store, and did not charge me for his "examination" and his advice. I invited him to talk to my class about the qualities of his work that make him a professional. Here are the highlights:

[Being a professional means having] technical ability and knowing where to go to get the answers. What you don't know, you'll continue to learn. The real professionals take the challenges. . . . Updating the client, discussing options . . . integrity, going for the customer's greatest good even though it may not be what they want. If what they want leaves them with an unsafe car because they won't allow me to fix something essential, then I won't work on it. . . . Accountability: If you make mistakes, it's essential that you are up-front. . . . Diagnosis is finding out what's right, which helps finding out what's wrong. . . . Having joy in your work, which is infectious, inspires other people, converts problems into opportunities.

His closing words of wisdom: "Unless you are all of this, you'll get a lot of one-time customers."

A public relations expert who once worked for a hospital consortium also spoke to the class. She described her work as "a researcher, teacher, facilitator, nudger, writer, and advocate . . . as if I have a desk in every hospital." She said,

Communication is two-way. It doesn't work without feedback. Integrity and honesty are much more important than saying what they want to hear. . . . My job is to elevate the clients to think about the greater good. . . . I get joy from watching the light bulbs go off, when my clients and I are sitting around the table. . . . Being a professional is being comfortable giving away my ideas, like a teacher.

The president of a small recording company talked about

all the experiences that I drew upon to be where I am, jobs that I had that I didn't like . . . a passion for doing what I do. . . . I juggle many connections. . . . I work with people around me who love what they do. . . . I want to present music with honesty and integrity. . . . I've had to learn to negotiate relationships that reflect honesty and integrity. . . . I learn new things about an industry from doing what I do every day. I'm learning all the time.

A public relations consultant talked about connections. When a potential client called him with a project outside his area of expertise, he told the client that he would connect with someone who knew the field. His client asked that he oversee the project, even though he was not doing the actual work, because he recognized that the consultant would be his advocate.

Another speaker used to be an international "pork jobber," a middleman connecting sellers with manufacturers. But he also made other sorts of connections. He used his knowledge of the market's potential to make recommendations to manufacturers about their assembly-line layouts. He came up with new ideas enabling slaughterhouses to use pork parts they usually discarded. He applied what he had learned in new creative ways.

All of these people are "professionals." Some, like the auto mechanic, had specific technical training. The public relations man and the pork jobber learned much of their skill on the job. They all combine many professional qualities: They are reliable and trustworthy; they neutralize any potential conflicts of interest with their integrity. They communicate well and help their clients understand. They are self-critical, collaborate with others, and know their limitations. They oversee and advocate for their clients in complex situations. They look at problems in new ways and come up with original ideas. They create new connections between people and between ideas. They see additional opportunities that can benefit their clients. They are *experienced*; that is, they not only have an awareness of similar situations from their professional lives, but they are also sufficiently reflective to know what can go wrong and what to anticipate. They are passionate about their work; they get joy from it. They work to build relationships with their clients; without the relationships, they would be less effective.

A professional's skills are transferable from one setting to another. The president of one corporation can move into a completely different setting with ease and use her insights and experience; all she needs is to learn the issues peculiar to the new position. And sometimes it even helps to have come from a different field, for then she can take a new, original, and creative look at the new situation. And so it is not surprising that the pork peddler is now a hospital chaplain, and the recording company executive used to be a schoolteacher.

PROFESSIONAL QUALITIES OF THE PHYSICIAN

What qualities, beyond technical knowledge and skill, define the physician as professional? Consider this complex medical history.

Following a neck injury that had caused arm weakness from pressure on his spinal cord, a 42-year-old man had cervical spine fusion surgery and was placed in a neck brace to immobilize his neck while it healed. Two days after surgery, he became confused. The nurse thought that his confusion might be related to the intravenous morphine being used for pain control. The neurosurgeon arranged for internal medicine consultation. The internist explored possible causes of the confusion by reading the hospital chart, reviewing the story with the patient and his wife, examining the patient, and performing a number of tests.

The internist stopped the morphine and corticosteroid medication, the other possible drug-related cause of his confusion, and the confusion cleared. But soon afterward, the patient had a respiratory arrest, probably related to aspiration of stomach contents into the lungs, and he required use of a mechanical ventilator for several days. When the ventilator was discontinued, he had difficulty swallowing. The neurosurgeon speculated that the swallowing difficulty was related to swelling of the upper airway from the intubation following surgery, but he realized that he had not previously seen this complication under quite these circumstances. The internist and the neurosurgeon agreed to obtain a neurological consultation.

For the neurologist, this was also a unique situation. She reviewed the history with the patient and his wife, read the hospital chart, examined the patient, and discovered several neurological findings suggesting cranial nerve deficit and abnormal brainstem function. She reviewed the medical literature. She called the internist to discuss the case and then ordered a specialized x-ray study (an MRI) of the brainstem and the upper spinal cord.

The MRI confirmed the neurologist's conclusions. She felt that no specific drug or surgical treatment was necessary, for she anticipated almost complete spontaneous recovery. The patient received a temporary feeding tube in order to avoid further aspiration from swallowing and continued with the neck brace and physical therapy.

During this illness, the patient and his wife became increasingly frustrated, angry, and depressed. Throughout that time, the internist provided them with information, interpretation, and emotional support.

Following discharge from the hospital, the patient saw the neurologist periodically to assess his swallowing and muscle function and the neurosurgeon to check
on the healing of his surgical wound. The patient and his wife continued to see the
internist at one- to two-month intervals.

A step-by-step review of the history provides many insights about the
physician as professional. Returning to the history:

Following a neck injury that had caused arm weakness from pressure on his spinal
cord, a 42-year-old man had cervical spine fusion surgery and was placed in a neck
brace to immobilize his neck while it healed. Two days after surgery, he became
confused. The nurse thought that his confusion might be related to the intravenous morphine being used for pain control. The neurosurgeon arranged for internal medicine consultation.

Professionals have excellent technical skills. Neurosurgeons know how to
diagnose spinal cord injury and do the corrective surgery. Internists know
how to address the differential diagnosis of confusion, how to treat it, and
ways to help prevent it from reoccurring. Some skills overlap.

Professionals know how quickly and urgently a problem needs to be treated.
Most neck injuries do not require emergency treatment. Those with neurological deficits, such as the arm weakness, may require urgent intervention
to prevent permanent disability.

Professionals define the issues and know how to manage them. Unless we use
our knowledge, experience, wisdom, and common sense, we cannot adequately address all the important issues. These issues are equally essential to
the *process* of care as to insuring the best possible *outcome.* In the case described, we cannot overlook treatable causes of confusion and swallowing
difficulty or neglect the human side of care.

*Professionals know their limitations and when to call for help, and recognize that
medicine is a collaborative profession.* They recognize their personal strengths and
limitations. They realize that a whole community of support is available and
are at ease taking useful suggestions, even from patients.

Professionals know how to move efficiently within the system. They know the
inner workings of the hospital and how to get things done quickly. When
they hit a snag, they know whom to call. Like a good mechanic, they know
the tricks of the trade. Like the savvy military noncommissioned officer
who has been around for a while, they know how to get around the rules
that get in the way. When the patient asks for another opinion, professionals not only accede to the request but call to get a timely appointment, pass
on the pertinent information, and make sure that the patient gets what he
or she needs.

The internist explored possible causes of the confusion by reading the hospital chart, reviewing the story with the patient and his wife, examining the patient, and performing a number of tests.

Professionals look at problems in more than one way and are flexible in their approach. They see beyond the apparent confines of a problem to define it accurately and solve it. They approach decisions about diagnosis and treatment carefully and consider all the possible alternatives; they do not jump to conclusions. Though the solutions to most medical problems are straightforward, some require real creativity. Professionals do not confine their diagnostic thoughts to the data at hand and go beyond the apparent boundaries defined by the history, physical findings, time intervals, and preconceptions to define the problem completely. Real professionals eschew an inappropriately narrow point of view for one that is flexible and creative.

And so in this case, the internist did not prematurely conclude that the confusion was drug related. Instead, he asked, "What are the possible causes of confusion in this postoperative patient, who is on intravenous feedings and had a long anesthesia?" He came up with this differential diagnosis:

- Drug-induced illness, from morphine or corticosteroids—and so he stopped them.
- Stroke—and so he did a neurological examination.
- Pneumonia—and so he examined the patient's lungs and obtained a chest x-ray.
- An electrolyte disturbance—and so he checked the concentration of blood electrolytes.
- A disorder of the acid-base level—and so he checked the blood pH.
- Hypoxemia (low oxygen level)—and so he checked the blood gas levels.
- Hypoglycemia—and so he checked the blood sugar.
- Anemia—and so he checked the hemoglobin.
- A "silent" myocardial infarct, one without symptoms—and so he examined his heart and checked the EKG.

All of the examinations and tests were normal. While the nurse's conclusion that the confusion was drug related was correct, the physician had to explore other diagnostic possibilities to answer the question, "What's the cause of the confusion?" lest another treatable cause be overlooked. *Professionals know what can go wrong and what questions to ask.*

The internist stopped the morphine and corticosteroid medication, the other possible drug-related cause of his confusion, and the confusion cleared. But soon afterward, the patient had a respiratory arrest, probably related to aspiration of stomach contents into the lungs, and he required use of a mechanical ventilator for several days. When the ventilator was discontinued, he had difficulty swallowing. The neurosurgeon speculated that the swallowing difficulty was related to swelling of the upper airway from the intubation following surgery, but he realized that he had not previously seen this complication under quite these circumstances. The internist and the neurosurgeon agreed to obtain a neurological consultation.

For the neurologist, this was also a unique situation. She reviewed the history with the patient and his wife, read the hospital chart, examined the patient, and discovered several neurological findings suggesting cranial nerve deficit and abnormal brainstem function. She reviewed the medical literature. She called the internist to discuss the case and then ordered a specialized x-ray study (an MRI) of the brainstem and the upper spinal cord.

Professionals know how to use the literature of medicine, including the textbooks and journals, *and how to use the medical librarian as a consultant* in the search for information.

Professionals use routines that allow for clear and precise thinking in the face of problems never previously encountered. Routines usually lead to the precise definition of the problem and the remedy, even with problems we have never encountered. Part of our professional training is learning such routines. Even though she had no previous experience with a problem exactly like this one in exactly the same setting, the neurologist fell back on a professional "routine" as she asked:

- What is the name of the problem? She called it "dysphagia" or difficulty swallowing.
- Where is the disease? Where in the body might the cause be? She considered a problem with the esophagus, but neurologic examination placed it in the site of the cranial nerve roots in the brainstem.
- What specific disease process could affect the brainstem in this way? A blood clot causing permanent brainstem damage (stroke) and ischemia (temporary diminished blood flow to the brainstem causing temporary damage) were most likely.
- What are the treatment choices? Of those, what is the best choice? Allowing time to elapse without specific treatment seemed to be the best course.

She called the internist to discuss the case and then ordered a specialized x-ray study (an MRI) of the brainstem and the upper spinal cord.

Professionals recognize that collaboration is an ongoing process. In their discussion, the internist and the neurologist questioned each other, added information, critiqued their hypotheses, and talked about the prognosis for the various causes of the brainstem abnormality, and only then did they proceed with the complex test. As a collaborative team, the neurosurgeon, internist, and neurologist knew what could go wrong and recognized the obligation to seek and offer advice. They also recognized that someone had to oversee the whole process and decided on the internist. An uncoordinated case runs the risk of mismanagement.

The MRI confirmed the neurologist's conclusions. She felt that no specific drug or surgical treatment was necessary, for she anticipated almost complete spontaneous recovery. The patient received a temporary feeding tube in order to avoid further aspiration from swallowing and continued with the neck brace and physical therapy.

During this illness, the patient and his wife became increasingly frustrated, angry, and depressed. Throughout that time, the internist provided them with information, interpretation, and emotional support.

Following discharge from the hospital, the patient saw the neurologist periodically to assess his swallowing and muscle function and the neurosurgeon to check on the healing of his surgical wound. The patient and his wife continued to see the internist at one- to two-month intervals.

Professionals try to minimize the chaos. They do this by approaching the sum of the problems and the patient and family in a systematic way. What was supposed to have been a straightforward hospitalization for this patient—surgery, a week's postoperative care, and discharge home—became chaotic. By interpreting all the information to the patient and his family, *professionals provide an integrated message, reassurance, and moral support.* Even when there are no treatments to alter or tests to monitor, periodic encounters help to identify and address the patient's and the family's concerns and uncertainties. The internist became the final conduit of information to the patient and his wife.

Professionals are consistent in their demeanor. Regardless of whom we see or when we see them, we do not allow our mood to intrude on the transaction. We are the same.

Professionals treat each patient and family member respectfully. We help the patient and family through all the steps and transitions of an illness and recognize that each member of the family may have a different view of the illness and a different relationship with the patient.

Professionals neutralize conflicts of interest. As professionals, we do not take financial advantage of our patients. Our patients' needs are primary. Even though we may earn a larger fee by providing a more expensive service, we do only what is appropriate, no more, no less. The surgeon operates only when indicated. The gastroenterologist does a procedure only when it adds to the solution. The psychiatrist sees a patient for neither too few sessions nor too many. Like my auto mechanic, the physician may well forgo a fee when a patient comes in with an obvious problem—a skin lesion that needs to be removed, a severe sprain—for which she would have to be referred elsewhere, even though he spends time and gives careful thought to considering the problem.

Professionals know how to talk to patients and their families in understandable language. We know that absent effective communication, the transaction is far more difficult.

Professionals are the patient's advocate. In many ways, the internist was this patient's advocate, moving the progress of his case along. He was skeptical about explaining away the swallowing difficulty as a result of the endotracheal tube; he suggested neurological consultation when the cause was unclear. He took the initiative to oversee the overall care of the patient once he had left the hospital. He helped the patient and his wife with their choices. When he involved consultants, he oversaw their work.

Professionals make connections. We connect with consultants. We connect our experience with new situations and transfer what we learned from one context to another. We connect information and ideas. We see connections between problems, how the coexistence of two illnesses can modify the choices of treatment, and how a treatment for one illness can adversely affect the course of a coexisting illness. We deal with many problems simultaneously.

Professionals think ahead. We know what can go wrong. We know how to minimize surprises.

Professionals know how to validate and critique their own work. We ask, "Are my decisions haphazard, or do I draw on the lessons of my experience? What could I have done differently?" We are willing to admit that we have made a mistake. We are always learning.

"*A professional is someone who can do his best work when he doesn't feel like it,*" wrote novelist James Agate.[1] We may not feel like it when we are tired, when we are troubled by something that is going on in our personal life, and even when we do not like our patient.

And finally, *faced with a difficult problem or a difficult patient, master professionals say, "This is fascinating."*

JUDGMENT

Professionals use judgment, a very special quality. A cardiologist taught it this way in a course on how to select patients for coronary bypass surgery.

A 50-year-old man, a nonsmoker in otherwise good health, had recurring chest pain. A cardiac stress test was positive. Coronary angiogram showed areas of narrowing in all three arteries. "How many of you would recommend bypass surgery?" the teacher asked. Everyone raised a hand. "Now let me change the circumstances," he continued. "Suppose he is 80 and smokes ten cigars a day. How many of you would recommend surgery for this man?" Nobody voted for the surgery. "We operated on George Burns two months ago and he has made a nice recovery." [Burns, of course, was the venerable cigar-smoking comedian who lived and worked for another twenty years.]

While rules of thumb—no heart surgery after a certain age, no surgery on smokers—are helpful guides, they are only a beginning. As we look more carefully at each patient as an individual, we learn to characterize the patient more precisely so that we can make important distinctions. Perhaps Burns got special consideration because of his celebrity, but that celebrity opened the door to more thoughtful consideration. Is age an absolute criterion, or should we consider someone's intellect, productivity, vitality, and connections to family? Does smoking absolutely contraindicate the surgery when the risks of no treatment are greater? Judgment involves knowing when to ask such questions and how to discover the answers.

Experience refines judgment. Judgment involves attention to details, the "total of little things,"[2] and integration of those details into clinical decisions. Practicing medicine is not like following a cookbook. Here are some other instances where judgment is important:

- When a patient has gallstones and recurring abdominal pain: Gallstones do not always cause pain, and often no test answers the questions, "Are the gallstones causing the pain? Does the patient need surgery?" The physician has to decide.

- When a person has recurring back pain for many years, and in the last week the pain has changed in intensity: The physician has to decide whether this change is more of the same or whether he has to search for an additional illness, such as cancer, to explain the change.

- When a 40-year-old man has angina: Even though there is no real emergency, the physician has to decide whether to expedite the tests, because delaying the tests will prolong the patient's anxiety.

- When screening blood tests show some unanticipated abnormality and the patient has neither symptoms nor objective signs of illness: The physician has to decide whether to go further.

Judgment is more than intuition. It involves integration of the history, the physical examination, the tests, the clinical context, and the psychosocial elements. Judgment involves looking at things in more than one way and testing them intellectually. Professionals know that there may be many possible answers. How we look at the essence of medicine—problems, relationships, interactions between medical problems, diagnosis, treatment, and prognosis—requires an open mind and an ongoing urge to ask, "Is there another way to look at this?" The more closely we analyze the elements of judgment, the better we can teach it.

Of the myriad judgments physicians make, one of the most important is deciding whether the patient has a serious illness.

A 32-year-old woman saw her physician because of headaches, recurring over several months. They occurred only on weekdays, were not associated with other neurological symptoms, and had gotten worse coincident with the uncertainties of the relationship with her boyfriend. Her physical examination was normal. Her physician tentatively concluded she needed no further tests. The next step was to address the psychosocial issues. When she returned a month later, the headaches were gone.

Not only was it important to decide, promptly and tentatively, that the patient did not have a serious illness, it was equally important to address the psychosocial issues. Ignoring that dimension of her symptoms would have prolonged her headaches and squandered the opportunity to help her address what was going on in her life. All of this takes judgment.

So from whose standpoint—the patient's, the physician's, the third parties,' or all of theirs—should we address the question, "What does it mean that the physician is a professional?" Actually it is an integration of their concerns.

Surely, the system fails when it does not meet the patient's needs, but physicians cannot accede to patients' requests that are otherwise of dubious. With each interaction with patients and colleagues, physicians need to apply their professional standards. The third parties—hospitals, insurers, government, and related institutions—often have useful information for patients and physicians to consider: cost, impact on the community, unrecognized community needs, and effective and ineffective treatment. But the third parties' view is inappropriate when it dictates action that undermines professionals' values and patients' needs. And when there is tension, the remedy is to return to the axiom, "The patient is the center of the drama," and ask, "What more can I learn from this dilemma?"

The drama of the Apollo 13 spacecraft rescue helped me to clarify further the answer to "What is a professional?" As presented in the movie of the same name, the spacecraft was seriously damaged halfway to the moon, and the three astronauts' lives were in jeopardy. The problem was: Get them back alive using the available energy resources and equipment aboard the spacecraft. The solution drew on the expertise of many specialists. The new technology and equipment were important to their rescue, but they would have been useless without these timeless dimensions: defining the problem, using the available resources, collaboration among many experts, and someone to coordinate all of this and maintain morale. Wisdom, ingenuity, common sense, efficiency, and genuine collaboration saved the lives of the astronauts.

In the transaction between the New England doctor and the Yankee dowager mentioned earlier, what went wrong? How could it have been done better? What was "unprofessional"? Both of them lost. She lost a good doctor. He lost a patient who might have been interesting to know because he overlooked the importance of the packaging, presentation, and first impression. If a person is going to call himself "doctor," he should *act* like a doctor. First impressions *are* important. Whether we like it or not, that first impression tentatively defines us for many people. Later on, we fill in the picture. When I first meet a patient who is on "isolation precautions" in the hospital because of infection, I am careful to show him my entire uncovered face before I cover it with a mask and get on with my examination. In that way, he sees more of me than a fraction of who I am. When I first meet a new class in the informal college setting, I dress up. In that way, they get an impression of me as a physician; later on, I come to class dressed more casually.

Patients want to be able to say, "Here is someone who will take things in hand, who knows what she's doing." They want to feel comfortable that the physician will do neither too little nor too much. The professional qualities of the physician protect the patient far more than rules, laws, and authorization to sue. These qualities are neither hard to achieve for the physician nor optional. They are implicit in every interaction. They are part of the job. They are what good doctors do all the time. These professional values keep physicians interested, stimulated, excited about their work, and fascinated.

The next chapter examines values in greater depth.

Chapter 17

Values and Dealing with Change

"We define ourselves by the sum total of our moral choices."

Among the questions prospective physicians ask are, "How do we deal with two conflicting views of medicine? On the one hand, medicine is a stimulating, satisfying, and challenging career; on the other, medicine is an institution in the midst of great change and outside regulation. How do physicians deal with all the changes in medicine, where we have seen a transition from care by one physician to care divided among many specialists, nurses with greater skills, growth in technology, greater access by patients to information through the lay press and internet, involuntary shifts of patients from one physician to another because of insurance coverage, and less attention to the human side of medicine?" These are complex questions about values.[1]

The answers are based on a number of assumptions, among which are:

- A values-based professional career provides the opportunity for consistent and thoughtful practice and promotes the highest level of service. Early statements of values in medicine include the Hippocratic Oath and the Oath of Maimonides.[2] Students often write their own statements of values, and I have included one example at the end of this chapter.

- Values guide decisions, validate positions, and prevent ethical drift. Values help to protect patients from abuse.

- Change is a reality of our personal and professional lives. A values-based career helps to ensure professional satisfaction and cope with change.

Values influence physicians' decisions as much as their knowledge and experience. Attending to values enriches each clinical experience. When we have values against which to measure our actions, we can declare more easily, "I won't do that. It conflicts with my values." Consciously or unconsciously, values help to define the physician.

Ethical matters include patient autonomy, the right of patients to make their own decisions, the right to privacy, and the question of competence to make an informed decision. Clinical decisions must integrate the patient's values into diagnostic and therapeutic choices, for example, the choice between a mastectomy for cancer of the breast or a breast-preserving procedure (lumpectomy). And the physician's values must be integrated into choices, for example, physicians who cannot accede to a request to terminate a pregnancy because of religious convictions.

There are clinical decisions in which the patient's values conflict with the physician's, for example, the son who declares, "Do everything you can for my father," while the physician believes that attending solely to comfort is a better choice. There are decisions in which members of a family disagree among themselves, such as how to proceed with their parent's care. Values help to clarify differences and reasons for conflict.

There are clinical choices where rules by outside agencies must be integrated into clinical choices, for example, when a doctor declares, "I am unable to do this test [admit this patient to the hospital, make this referral, etc.] because the patient's medical plan doesn't allow it." There are choices regarding career tracks, such as suburban or inner city practice, primary care or a specialty.

And so the next question is, "What are the challenges to our values?"

Those considering a medical career or beginning as medical students are usually sensitive to the human needs of patients; often that is why medicine is so attractive to them. As they experience more intense patient contact, and certainly by the time they reach postgraduate medical residency training, time pressure and the message "Don't get too involved" often challenge that sensitivity.

The cost of *becoming* a physician is substantial, and recouping the cost may affect our choice of specialty or practice style. Financial issues can be a strong motivator, but if earning power were the only motivation, all doctors would choose high-earning specialties. They do not, because of skills and aptitude, length of training, the nature of the professional life—and values. One undergraduate saw that "compensation goes beyond wages. Intellectual and social benefits can be as attractive as economic compensation." Partly because of values, physicians choose to be internists or cardiac surgeons, to be a fulltime doctors or work three-quarters time, to practice in a city or a small town, to be home for dinner with the kids or not make it until much later.

We choose our style of practice on the basis of values. When I was a medical student, I heard this from more than one of my community-based teachers: "This is the way you do it in the medical center—the thorough way, spending time with each patient—but you can't do it this way once you're in practice." A colleague recently told me, "Whether a physician spends ten minutes or twenty with a patient will be market-driven." Insurance companies, managed care organizations, and other third-party payers sometimes dictate rules that have impact on everyday decisions: length of stay in the hospital, choice of referrals and tests, and length of time spent with a patient. Yet no more would we ask a surgeon to remove a portion of diseased bowel in fifteen minutes when it ordinarily takes more than an hour, than should we ask an internist to explore a patient's medical history in fifteen minutes, when it usually takes forty-five. Doing it the right way is essential to our integrity as doctors.

At the conclusion of Woody Allen's 1989 movie, *Crimes and Misdemeanors*, the character to whom he always returns says, "We are all faced with moral choices. . . . We define ourselves by the sum total of our moral choices." Here are some moral choices physicians make. They are actually statements of value.

- Always remember that the patient is the center of the drama.
- Pick the right place to practice. The location—small town or big city, the culture, and the values of the office and hospital setting—is just as important as the choice of specialty. The same physician can be unhappy and unfulfilled in one position and flourish in another. The same patient can feel alone and unattended by one physician and respected and truly cared for by another. From one of my teachers, not a physician, I learned, "Who you are depends on where you are."
- Maintain your sense of creativity. Do something new each year.
- Maintain your integrity.
- Do not hedge on time. The quality of the transaction depends on time.
- Devise a thoughtful integration of personal life and practice.
- Do not compromise. Responding to a question regarding "technically oriented" directors who "don't respect the actor's craft," actor Paul Newman once observed, "The pace never controls the actor, the actor controls the pace. The second that that happens [the pace and the director control the actor], the actor

loses his humanity."[3] The second that outside pressures begin controlling us as physicians, we lose *our* humanity.

Loss of humanity can occur not only in relation to patients but also in relation to our professional associates. I know of conflicts within partnerships, not over the quality of care the partners are providing, but rather over office logistics—and values. With tongue in cheek, one partner observed, "It's not the money, it's the money." I know of a physician who left a partnership because one of his associates, a technically competent doctor, treated patients and staff disrespectfully. I know of one who left a lucrative practice for another one less so because he felt devalued. He decided that even if he made less money, it was more important that he maintain his integrity.

The Illness Narratives by Arthur Kleinman provides good text for teaching about values.[4] It contains stories about eight contemporary physicians, each of whom has a different way of looking at patients, practice, and challenges. I ask my undergraduate students to describe how each approaches the challenges of practice. One junior wrote:

Each [physician] blends his/her personal beliefs, professional ideologies, cultural biases, individual personalities, and life philosophies to develop a role in the physician-patient relationship. One important characteristic is how the physician views the patient and views himself. Is the patient a "diseased patient," a "diseased person," or a "person with a disease"? Is the physician there to fight the disease? To fix the patient? Or to talk with the patient [about] what the problems are and find possible solutions? . . . [Physicians who] view the patient as a business transaction differ greatly from those who view the patient as a person in need. . . . Those who view being a physician as merely a daily routine respond to their patients very differently from those who view being a physician as a way of life.

I also ask, "How does each of these physicians deal with the dilemmas they face in medicine?" The student continued:

[In the text, the] young medical student . . . is unsure of his role and responsibilities as a physician. [He] feels great compassion and emotion for his dying patient. Although he realizes that the emotions are understandable, he fears that it may compromise the quality of his care. . . . [My hope is] he will realize that compassion and empathy are fundamental to a physician's care and do not conflict with providing efficient, quality care.

Of another physician described in the chapter, a sophomore wrote:

[He] deals with the dilemmas of medicine by tapping into his experiences as a patient and as someone who has felt the grief of losing a loved one. These feelings help him to better identify with the patient, thereby providing the kind of care that does not just deal with the patient's body, but with all aspects of his or her life. He immerses himself in his work, not only because of his love for what he does, but partly out of a need he feels to be effective. This need, in combination with his childhood experiences, helps to define how he deals with any dilemmas he may encounter in medicine.

A junior wrote, "I believe that each physician can incorporate his own personal value system into his practice. . . . What patient wouldn't prefer a physician interested in the caring and healing aspect of medicine over one whose ability is suffocated by legal and political facts?"

In a first-year course at the University of Minnesota, medical students also address questions of values. One constructed a personal mission statement with a set of values.

Above all, I will be a good husband and father. I will set aside time to spend with my immediate and extended family and my close friends and will help them whenever I can. . . . I will maintain balance between work and home. . . . I will remember that the patient is the center of the drama. I will always view patients as individuals rather than as cases. I will not make assumptions about patients; instead, I will listen to their stories. I will give culturally competent care. . . . I will remember that patients have very individual reactions and perspectives. . . . I will willingly teach others what I know. . . . I will scrutinize my actions for consistency with my beliefs and values. . . . I will answer for my mistakes.

A classmate observed:

In dealing with patients and families, honesty is as valuable as knowledge. No amount of medical education will teach a student to tell the truth and maintain professionalism while interacting with people, yet it remains [essential] to the practice of medicine. . . . It does not take a long time to tell the truth, just as it does not take an excessive amount of time to be a compassionate physician. . . . Almost all of the patients that we have met with this year have asked for the same basic things: If you don't know the answer to a question, don't make it appear as if you do. If you do know the answer to a question, be honest and present it in an appropriate manner. And, most importantly, listen. It makes the patient feel that you truly have a stake in their well being.

Undergraduates and beginning medical students get the picture: Their task is to maintain their values and to refine them. "How can I maintain my values in the face of all the outside pressures?" they ask. There are many ways.

Talk. Protect confidences certainly, but share stories, dilemmas, and values with a confidant, a peer, a life partner. Look to others, not necessarily physicians. Clergy, social workers, nurses, patients, and their families all have wisdom.

Listen. Listen carefully for clues to patients' values. Be aware that buried in what patients tell you may be important clues to *their* values, which may explain their struggles, clarify reasons for conflict with the physician and others, and give clues to the remedy.

Read. Read critically. Books, both nonfiction and fiction, and newspapers are filled with stories with value-laden issues.

Reflect. From colleagues, discussions, books, conferences, and after each encounter with patients and their families, ask, "What did I learn?" Look for meaning. Leave time for reflection.

Teach. When we teach, we need to think and express ourselves clearly, define ourselves and our values, and defend what we have to say. When we teach, we model behavior and enter into a relationship with students and yet another opportunity to learn.

Choose models, physicians you admire, and find out about them. We might surmise that since physicians do not talk about values in their day-to-day conversations, they do not think about them. Yet all the physicians who have spoken to my classes have been profound in their reflections, and each has presented a personal creed. An academic orthopedist who cares for patients with especially complex problems, oversees a residency program, and does research has these priorities: "my family, my work, and my health, both mental and physical." A family practice specialist talks about her quest "to help patients make sense of their lives" and the importance of "self-forgiveness for making mistakes."

For the physician, there is, in fact, an implied triad of roles: I am a professional; I am a physician; I am (insert your name). Each role implies certain values. A clear set of values leaves little room for compromises of time, resources, accessibility, or compassion. To the extent that any of these values are compromised, we should simply declare, "This won't do."

First-year medical students at the University of Minnesota Medical School each January go through a rite of passage, the White Coat Ceremony, as they start to see patients. The 2001 program for that ceremony stated, "The respect that society assigns to the physician is related to the professional values and responsibilities of this calling. The compassion, kindness, self-sacrifice, scientific expertise, ethics, humanity, and equanimity of future physicians require that these values be taught and modeled by us."

Each physician is a guardian of the values of the profession. The physician knows best the details and nuances of individual patients and their illnesses. As their advocates, physicians efficiently shepherd patients through the system. We protect them from unnecessary testing and treatment and also from frivolous intrusion by third parties. In a greater sense, we also protect ourselves from incremental drifts of values. And as the guardians of the values of the profession, we set examples and are models for students, colleagues, and hospital and office staff. The rules, the *real rules*, are the values. Not only do the values protect the patient, they safeguard the integrity of the physician.

In this context, a physician can look at change and see challenges and opportunities. We expect patients to adjust to change all the time—change in health, life expectancy, and other losses. Why should we not expect physicians to do the same? Change is a reality of medicine, just as it is of any career. Change is a reality of life.

In cases where care by one physician has been divided among many specialists, the opportunity arises to provide better care, as does the need for someone to coordinate that care. Where nurses have developed even greater skills, there is more opportunity for nurse-physician partnership, sharing of responsibility, and learning from each other. With growth in technology comes the opportunity to treat more precisely and preserve more lives and the responsibility to use the technology wisely without using it to replace careful thought and clinical judgment. Where patients have greater access to information through the lay press and the internet, there is the responsibility to provide them with interpretation and professional judgment. Where insurance coverage forces involuntary shifts of patients from one physician to another, there is the responsibility to reassert the importance of the doctor-patient relationship. And where there is less attention to the human side of medicine, there is the need to reclaim this dimension as essential to good care.

When students take all of these reflections and integrate them with their own observations, they begin to understand the many different ways to be a complete and fulfilled physician. Ultimately, that is the goal of addressing the question, "What's it like to be a physician?"

Chapter 18

Becoming a Physician: The Evolution of a Career

"Who you are depends on where you are."

Think of the beginning of a medical career as the time that we enter medical school, rather than the moment when the first paycheck as a practicing physician, teacher, or researcher arrives. Many transitions occur: from student to practitioner and teacher, from less experienced to more experienced, from novice to veteran, from smaller income to larger, from one place to another. Changes come in age, expectations, values, and character and in the profession and the world at large. New diseases are identified, and the technology and views of illness evolve. But for the most part, the catalogue of diseases and problems a physician deals with remains the same, and the human dimension is timeless.

One of my colleagues, whom I have known since he was an intern, told me one day, "I'm turning 50 and I see things differently now. At 40, I was building a practice and doing lots of surgery because that's what I do. Now I'm a physician first, who also does surgery. I had a family conference about a lady who's had eight surgical procedures over the last month. Her daughter said, 'Pa, since mother's had her stroke, she hasn't had a happy day. What are we doing all this for?'" Older and wiser, the surgeon saw questions and issues that he had not seen as a younger physician. Indeed, how we look at our practice can skew how we deal with issues and conduct ourselves, how happy we are, how likely we are to become disenchanted, and how well we deal with change. The evolution of our career takes place in parallel with the evolution of our personal life, its successes and losses, the maturing of relationships, the renewal of old interests and the development of new ones. We miss a lot without growth.

None of these scenarios approximates what really happens:

- You decide to become a doctor. You go to medical school and learn what you have to. You become a doctor. You start practice alone or join an already established office and remain there for the duration of your professional career. You practice for thirty to forty years. You cease practicing. End of story.
- You are a sensitive, altruistic person. You become a doctor. End of story.
- You cannot stand the sight of blood. You cannot deal with a patient with an incurable illness. You cannot deal with death. You decide to become a doctor, and you immediately learn to deal with all these matters. End of story.

Just as the brief history that began this book, the one about the physician with heart disease who had coronary bypass surgery, does not do justice to his real story, neither does any one of these "histories" adequately describe the path with many detours that a medical career takes. We learn skills, to be sure, but we also refine goals and values. We change homes, towns, and practice situations. In the course of a career, we enhance our knowledge, become wiser in how we deal with patients, and become more realistic in what we can do and what we can predict. We make countless decisions outside of the patient-oriented ones—about how we let our career affect our personal lives and about what, of all the pressing matters, is especially important.

I like what Chaim Potok wrote in *In The Beginning*. His first-person protagonist is a teacher.

All beginnings are hard.

I can remember hearing my mother murmur those words while I lay in bed with fever. "Children are often sick, darling. That's the way it is with children. All beginnings are hard. You'll be all right soon."

I remember bursting into tears one evening because a passage of Bible commentary had proved too difficult for me to understand. I was about nine years old at the time. "You want to understand everything immediately?" my father said. "Just like that? You only began to study this commentary last week. All beginnings are hard. You have to work at the job of studying. Go over it again and again."

The man who later guided me in my studies would welcome me warmly into his apartment and, when we sat at his desk, say to me in his gentle voice, "Be patient. . . . You cannot swallow all the world at one time."

I say it to myself today when I stand before a new class at the beginning of a school year or am about to start a new book or research paper: All beginnings are hard. . . . And sometimes I add what I have learned on my own: "Especially a beginning that you make by yourself. That's the hardest beginning of all."[1]

The first surgery I ever witnessed was a ritual circumcision. I was 20, a senior in college, and had already been accepted to medical school. I almost fainted. The sight of blood does not bother me anymore. I grew. I evolved. I got handy at dealing with these things, but not overnight. How we evolve as physicians—our initial choice to become a physician and then what kind of a physician and human being we will become—depends on at least three factors: personal experience, role models, and the communities to which we belong. Though they vary in influence at any given time, ultimately we derive our values and our character from all of them.

- *Personal experience.* Just like patients, physicians have things going on in their lives—illness, concerns regarding parents, children, and income, and the frustrations of living a complex adult life. A good doctor handles them in ways that do not intrude on interactions with patients, but she can also use the insights and wisdom gained from these experiences in dealing with patients. And so in their first assignment in my seminar, I ask students to reflect on an illness that they or a family member experienced, what it was like for them, what were the best and worst parts of the experience, and how they handled it. Finally I ask them, "What do you learn from reflecting on all of this?"
- *Models.* My formative view of a physician came from our family doctor. I ask students, "Who are your models?" They talk about parents, relatives, friends, physicians, and teachers and the qualities that they wish to emulate. Over time, we add to our list of models.
- *Communities.* As we identify more closely with a community, we begin to reflect the community's values. Nationality, religion, and socioeconomic group are among the more commonly defined communities, but there are others. The neighborhood, the town or city, the specific place of worship, the school, the community of physicians, medical students, or residents, and others are all sources of values.

THE EDUCATION OF A PHYSICIAN

Learning about the human side of medicine never ceases, nor does it have a precise beginning. But let us define the parts of a physician's education as what precedes medical school, then medical school and residency training, and what follows.

Before Medical School

These are some of the lessons I learned from reflecting on my undergraduate years.

Of organic chemistry and embryology, I remember benzene rings, the ortho-, para- and meta- positions, that "ontology recapitulates phylogeny," and something about the embryonic aortic arches and their relation to the persistence after birth of a patent ductus arteriosis, a congenital abnormality of the blood vessel architecture near the heart. Though I did not retain much else, I learned how to organize information and learn in a systematic way. I learned that the more I learned, the easier it was to retain it, because I had an increasingly more refined structure to which to connect the new information.

I do not remember much from my two years of philosophy except that they were about "meaning." Now I have an interest in spirituality, which some define as finding meaning in life's events. I often ask patients, "What does this illness mean to you?" and that question often leads to a discussion of their fears. Philosophy was also about values. Now, as a physician, I know the importance of values and that if we do not have a strong sense of values at the beginning of our career, then it is harder to learn and adopt those values somewhere in midcareer.

I do not recall much detail from my general psychology course. But now I am fascinated by the psychology of groups—of organizations, meetings, medicine, and communities. Sometimes I ask patients, "Who is your community?" in order to find out to whom they turn to for support in times of need. From my psychology course, I also remember this exercise: Connect all nine dots with four straight lines without lifting the pencil from the paper (Figure 18.1). The imaginary square around the dots does not define the limits of the solution: Go outside the square to perform the task (Figure 18.2). As a teacher, I use this exercise as a way to teach that good physicians need to think originally, to go beyond the obvious borders of a problem, to look at things in yet one more way in order to consider all the options to solving a problem.

I hardly remember anything from my world history course. I do remember that World War I did not begin, as I learned in high school, because someone assassinated the archduke of Austria. The story began much earlier, as nations laid plans and formed alliances for the conquest of Europe. It is like that in medicine. Patients may begin the story of their illness where they *think* it began. Our task is to explore the story more completely, for it may have begun long before. Developing the patient's story in this way pro-

Figure 18.1

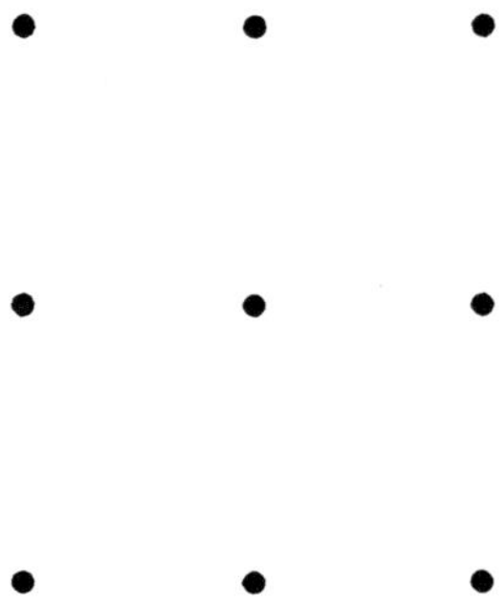

• • •

• • •

• • •

vides more insight into the illness and the patient's life, and it may influence the process of care and the outcome.

I started to study German as a freshman because I thought that German was the "language of science." I continued these studies because of the warm relationship I developed with my teacher of four years. Today, to develop the inquiry about the doctor-patient relationship, I often ask my students, "How is the doctor-patient relationship like the teacher-student relationship?" From my German teacher, I learned the importance of caring about a student—and saying so. Not a bad model for a teacher and a physician.

I have used the language with German-speaking patients, and because of my German training, I was able to hone my facility with Yiddish, a similar language and the language of Eastern European Jews. I had many opportunities to use it in speaking with Russian Jewish immigrants who became my patients. My interest in using their language enhanced our relationship. It is a good metaphor for the doctor-patient relationship: In order for the relationship to be a good one, the doctor needs to speak the patient's language, נאָך װי װײַ

As a senior I took a course in linguistics with only three other students. For one of our assignments, we were given a text of Swahili and the translation of a few words and asked to construct a Swahili grammar. Suddenly a light went on! I could do the task pretty comprehensively, evolving rule after rule, testing the newly evolved rule with another part of the text. For me, this was a major step in deductive and creative reasoning, the result of an active partnership with my teacher. Deductive and creative reasoning and partnership between the patient and the doctor are a large part of medicine.

In my freshman English seminar, I learned to write and to express myself clearly. To do that, I needed to organize and clarify my thoughts, critique and edit myself, and internalize what my professor did for me so that I could become my own teacher. In four years of required public speaking courses, I

Figure 18.2

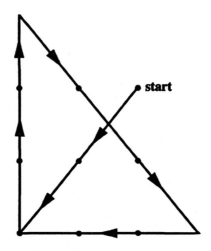

learned to make my presentation more interesting; that skill comple-
mented my ability to write. As a physician and teacher, I choose my words
carefully. I ask myself, "What works and what doesn't? Did my patient or
my student hear it as I meant it?" When I was in practice, I "edited" my patients' stories, taking their spontaneous narratives and turning them into
cohesive wholes without altering the sense and the facts, so that I could
draw valid conclusions and communicate clearly with my colleagues. Now
students are my audience, and I tell them that part of the way I evaluate
them is by their ability to write and speak. Physicians need to think, speak,
and write clearly.

But I did not learn much about choosing a career in college. I never
looked carefully at myself, my values and choices, how I would integrate my
personal and my professional life, and what it was *really* like to be a physician. Though I have never regretted my choice of professions, if I had
known better, I would have chosen more deliberately. I try to help my undergraduate students make an informed choice.

Now, in retrospect, I appreciate my undergraduate years more and more,
and I know:

- An undergraduate education is a gem, a once-in-a-lifetime opportunity to prepare, in the broadest sense, for a career; to look at our abilities and aptitudes, priorities, and personality; and to define and refine our values. After all, among the
  most important choices in life is that of a career and life's work.

- There are seeds of insight being planted in each of the courses undergraduates
  take. Their task as perpetual students is to recognize these insights. Students

need not be concerned if they do not see them yet, for they may become apparent only years later. One simply needs an open, inquiring mind.

- As teachers, it is our special task to transmit not simply information but techniques for learning and how to inquire. We need to help students frame or reframe their questions. We need to keep as open and inquiring as we ask our students to be. We need to know how to be good models. And we need to learn from our students.

The years before medical school provide many lessons and insights about the human side of medicine as well as endless opportunities to learn and reflect. People sensitive to the human issues emerge from different paths: science majors and those majoring in music, engineering students and those expert in history, people right out of college and those starting medicine one or a few years later, often as a second career. All have in common intellectual capacity and curiosity, a commitment to lifelong learning, and the human qualities.

Medical School and Residency

How do we preserve the sensitivity to the human side of medicine that most bring to medical school? How do we maintain the values we have defined from our experience, models, and community? If medical students begin with all this wisdom and sensitivity, what happens to it? During medical school and residency, we learn skills in diagnosis, treatment, and prognosis and we refine those skills—at a minimum. What about the human side?

No small part of a career in medicine are the years in medical school and residency. If our professional life is the sum of four years of medical school, three to six years or more of residency training, and thirty years of practice, then medical school and residency constitute up to a fourth of our professional life; and so prospective doctors ought to know what it is like. I have heard descriptions ranging from "exhilarating and wonderful" to "dehumanizing and awful." What makes it different for each person has to do with preparation, clarity of purpose, wisdom in parsing out our life to school and the rest of our life, how we deal with stress, and how well we learn.

Choosing the right medical school and residency helps us preserve our humanity. Students often choose on the basis of quality and cost, but beyond those factors, they often consider:

- The "culture" of the place, what it is like to be there. Is it an atmosphere that supports its students in their process of learning, recognizes them as individuals, models the relationship with patients, addresses values, and endorses and teaches the biopsychosocial model of medicine? Does it teach what it is like to be a professional? What are the students like? Is the atmosphere collegial or "cut-throat?" Is there an *esprit de corps* among the students? Are students at ease talking about their insecurities and failures as well as their successes? Is there recognition of diversity among the student body and the body of patients—ethnic and national diversity, marital status, sexual orientation? Does the school pay attention to their individual needs? What are the forces that may subtly and incrementally alter their innate sensitivity and values?

- The location. Where is the medical school or residency program located? Big city or small town? Do the qualities of the community—ethnic makeup, cultural offerings—meet the needs of the physician-in-training? For those who are single and looking for a life's partner, what are the possibilities? For those with a family, what does the community offer?

"Institutions cultivate what they honor,"[2] a colleague has said. When medical schools and residency programs teach the human side of medicine as an essential component of training, throughout the curriculum, modeled and practiced by its physician-teachers, then those programs indeed support, refine, and reinforce the humanity the student brings. But when the human side is taught haphazardly and sporadically, with leftover time, then students can begin to question its worth. Time can be a barrier. Programs must allocate time to teach, model, and practice the human side. More and more medical schools and residency programs are devoting adequate time to address and teach these issues. I encourage my students to seek out those places.

After Residency

Times change, along with information, technology, and interests. Changes affect what we do as physicians and where. Changing where we practice is not unusual as a career evolves. Some physicians, even without moving, have altered their practice situation to spend more time with their families. Physicians teach, lecture, advise, mentor, and write during their active professional years and thereafter, and they volunteer in health projects for the underprivileged at home and in third world countries. Many physicians are fine musicians.

Being a physician requires a commitment to lifelong learning. Even the timeless part of medicine, the human side, requires growth as we learn better strategies for speaking with patients and relating to them. Beyond the formal settings are the daily teachable moments with patients and colleagues and sources outside of medicine.

Being a physician provides many opportunities for doing something new. In the process of arranging a program of lectures and support for the staff of a nursing home many years ago, I asked a busy physician-teacher, the dean of St. Paul psychiatrists, to suggest some names of those who would lead such a program. "*I'll* do it," he said. "I always like to do something new each year." Hardly any profession provides as many opportunities to learn and to grow.

In dealing with stress, competence helps. Having an adequate fund of knowledge and knowing how to apply it appropriately minimize the number of stressful situations. When they do arise, it helps to ask, "What is this all about?" and "What can I learn?" Both questions liberate. It helps to have a confidant—a close friend, co-professional, peer, or life partner—with whom to share problems and feelings. Sometimes it is actually better to talk it over with a nonphysician who sees things differently.

Then there is the camaraderie with others in the healing professions—physicians, nurses, social workers, clergy, and other hospital and office staff—and the joy of collaborating with them, of teaching and learning from these validating peers and kindred spirits. "[When a physician] spends hour upon hour with people [i.e., patients] in whose company he has to efface his own needs, . . . he begins to feel a powerful need to be in the company of his colleagues, to exchange experiences, to learn, to feel secure, to obtain encouragement and support, even to hear objective criticism: to feel a sense of belonging to a framework, a tradition backing his work."[3] A doctor connects with very interesting people.

How we integrate our personal and professional lives varies. Sometimes there is simply no choice—the emergency that the on-call physician, the only doctor in town, or the only plastic surgeon around must handle. Then professional duty takes precedence over personal matters. But where there is a choice, where a physician is one of many, then we have the opportunity to define and act upon our priorities. There is life outside of medicine.

Physicians make different choices. Some consistently work well into the evening; others stop taking new patients when they find their practice is too busy. Some work less than fulltime. More and more, physicians are trimming their practice hours in order to spend more time with their families. I know of a surgeon who spends a day a week at a monastery. When he declined to run for reelection to the U.S. Senate after his diagnosis of lymphoma, the late Paul Tsongas declared: "No one on his death bed ever said, 'I wish I had spent more time with my business.'" What kind of physician we choose to become—not simply what specialty but also how we conduct our professional life and shape our career—has a great deal to do with our values. Part of many physicians' routine is periodically asking the strategic questions: "Where do I want to be in the next year? In five years? Have I stuck to my values?" A medical career provides the opportunity to fashion a life's work that meets our needs. A friend taught me, "Who you are depends on where you are."

A medical career is privileged in many ways. Among them are stimulation from the beginning to the end, the variety of ways to serve, and the opportunity to change and grow in ways that maintain our values and preserve the joy of the career.

PART III

THE DOCTOR-PATIENT
RELATIONSHIP

Chapter 19

The Qualities of the Doctor-Patient Relationship

"For as long as it takes."

If, as Shakespeare wrote, "All the world's a stage,"[1] and if each encounter between a patient and a physician is a drama, great or small, and if the patient is the center of the drama, then from these simple premises flow a number of inferences:

- Patients need help. If they could handle or solve their problems alone, using their own resources, they would not have come to the physician. In order to help, physicians must be certain to define the problem correctly.
- The physician must speak the patient's language, not vice versa. What physicians say to patients must be comprehensible.
- The physician must start where the patient is, not the other way around. Attending to this simple principle—an axiom of the social work profession—guides the entire transaction and keeps the process centered on the patient.
- The patient's needs are to be met, not the physician's, though doctors need to be happy in their work.
- The patient's problems are the subject of the transaction. They are not interested in hearing a parallel story from the physician's life.
- Patients could not care less whether theirs is an "interesting case."

What the physician does with the information obtained about the patient—the history, physical examination, and ancillary data—is process. Ultimately the results of this process come back to the transaction between the patient and the physician. And so it is worthwhile to describe the doctor-patient relationship in depth. It is not simply "being nice to the patient."

If you doubt that the relationship has importance, think of this: The relationship allows the physician to do painful things—press down hard on a really painful abdomen, for instance—without retaliation. It allows intimate examination—an examination of the rectum, pelvis, or breasts—without cries of assault. Think also about these questions:

- If there were just a few things that doctors could do that were *really* effective before the early twentieth century, when there was a real acceleration of technology and availability of effective drugs and other kinds of therapy, how come people went to doctors back then?

- If the relationship is important to the outcome of the illness, to the patient, and to the patient's family, could we do without it?

- What do physicians do when they have done nothing concrete; that is, they have not given the patient a prescription or done a procedure?

In the previous chapters, I have described in detail what it is like to be a patient and to be a physician. What does each bring to the doctor-patient encounter? Patients bring:

- Their needs and fears. What to the physician may be a self-limited illness with a good prognosis—abdominal pain from gastroenteritis, for instance—may mean to the patient that he has cancer. It is up to the physician to discover those fears of discomfort, uncertainty, and outcome.

- Their experiences. If encounters with other physicians have turned out well, their expectations will be similar for the current one, and they will likely be at ease. But if their experiences have been unpleasant or inconsistent, if prior physicians have been moody, unavailable, and incomprehensible, it will be no wonder that the patient may be tentative, suspicious, and argumentative.

- Their prejudices, positive and negative. "What kind of name is yours?" someone with positive or negative expectations of an ethnic group, race, gender, or manner of dress may ask. Dislikes based on prejudice may not last once time enriches the relationship, but such impressions may overpower the initial encounter.

- Their unstated agendas. "I'm here for an examination before my knee surgery" may disguise the concern that "this means I'm getting older and beginning to fall apart." A simple question from the physician, "What does this surgery mean to you?" can expose these fears.

- Their goals and expectations. "I want to be completely healed" may be the unspoken goal, or "I just want to make it to my daughter's wedding. Then I'll be content."

- Their values and those of the communities to which they belong.

- Their strengths and resources or lack thereof. They carry with them the knowledge of the ways they have met adversity and the successful strategies they used to solve them. They bring the experiences and examples of family and friends. "When my mother was ill with cancer, she handled it in an admirable way by. . . ." They bring the support of family and friends and their religion or philosophy of life.

To the encounter, physicians bring:

- Their credential, M.D., their technical expertise, and their humanity.

- Their prior professional experiences. After all, the reason the patient has come to a physician is because the doctor is *experienced* in dealing with such problems; the patient is not.

- Their prejudices. Though physicians ought to be prejudice-free, many are not. At the very least, though, they need to recognize their prejudices and neutralize them during the doctor-patient encounter.

- Consistency. Not "hot" one day and "cold" the next. Though the patient may be volatile and labile from one encounter to the next, the physician is consistent and therefore trustworthy. "I am the same. I will never lie to you. I will not abandon you," are the unspoken reassuring messages of this consistency.

- Calm at a time of upset, dismay, and uncertainty for the patient.

- Their own special strengths. Beyond the broad physician credential, they may be known for their expertise in a specialty, a subspecialty, or a particular illness, or their ability to listen, address the needs of the elderly or the rebellious teenager, or see the patient in the broad biopsychosocial context.

- What they have learned from life. As with the patient, there is more to physicians' lives than time spent in professional encounters. Successes and failures are potentially intrusive—for good or bad—on professional lives.

- Their values and those of the communities to which they belong, just as with patients. They are members of the medical community, to be sure, but they also may have religious values, "midwestern values" (in my own case), or others that flavor the way they treat patients.

- Fears. Of death, of making a mistake, and of failure.

Two generations ago, the most common model of a doctor-patient relationship was a paternalistic one: The physician told the patient, "This is what's wrong, and this is what you should do." Not much was negotiable. Implied was, "The doctor knows best." A far more acceptable model is "the enhanced autonomy model"[2] in which the patient and the physician are partners. There are no directives from the doctor to the patient; rather, there is an ongoing negotiation, integrating data, diagnosis, treatment options, and values. "Let's come to an understanding of what's going on. Let's both be sure we're reasoning from the same information. Let's be sure we have the same goals. Let me tell you what I think and then we'll negotiate." Most patients appreciate this approach.

Whatever the medical issues, the success of the transaction ultimately depends on the quality of the relationship between the physician and the patient. As we sharpen our ability to characterize that relationship, we can learn from our successes and mistakes, make use of our insights, and teach what we do.

Compare these two decisions (Table 19.1):

- Decision A. Whether to have an appendectomy for acute appendicitis, an acute illness for which surgery is almost always the only treatment and is almost always effective. Even in the elderly patient with many chronic illnesses, the chance of a bad outcome is small.

- Decision B. Whether to have palliative chemotherapy for breast cancer with widespread metastases. "Palliative" means that the treatment will not cure the illness; it may only delay its progression. Certain types of chemotherapy have substantial adverse side effects: nausea, loss of appetite, hair loss, and other organ toxicity. With chemotherapy, often there are no guarantees of success.

What is the role of the physician? How important is the relationship between the patient and the physician?

For the patient with appendicitis, the transaction is simple, involving few uncertainties. The outcome with treatment is almost always good. On the other hand, the patient with the malignancy needs ongoing physician involvement, understanding, inquiry into her values, and recognition that the decision to accept or reject the chemotherapy is not irrevocable. It is insufficient for the doctor to say, "Here are your choices. Take your pick." Over the duration of the illness, the physician provides validation, support, and the promise of future availability and keeps the patient from unnecessary or futile procedures. For the series of transactions to be most effective, they need a relationship.

Table 19.1
Comparison of Some Qualities of Appendicitis and Metastatic Breast
Cancer

Qualities	Appendicitis	Metastatic breast cancer
Without treatment		
• Outcome	Poor	Poor
• Level of uncertainty regarding outcome	Small	Small (will get worse)
With treatment		
• Outcome	Good	Variable
• Level of uncertainty regarding outcome	Small (will improve)	Substantial
• Duration of treatment	Short	Long
• Morbidity*		
• Duration of discomfort	Short	Long
• Level of discomfort	Small	Variable
Importance of patient's values in making decisions	Usually not important	Important
Need for long-term physician follow-up	Small	Substantial

*Morbidity: Duration and severity of the illness

If the prognosis is poor, then the relationship is especially important in sustaining the patient and family for the duration of the illness. Even when "nothing more can be done"—that is, no further treatment specific for the cancer—there is plenty more to do. The physician provides comfort, support, perspective, and interpretation.

Empathy is a primary quality of the relationship. A rabbi told me this story, one of my favorites: Two boys, the son of a rabbi and his best friend, decide to play a game. "You be the rabbi," says the son of the rabbi, "and I'll be his congregant." "Rabbi," the "congregant" says, "I'm having trouble in my marriage, trouble with my boss, and trouble with my daughter." Replies the "rabbi," "You should pay more attention to your wife, confront your boss, and make peace with your daughter." To which the rabbi's son replies, "No, no, no, you didn't do it right. You didn't first say, 'Oy!' "

I reminded myself of the story often while I was in practice. As a less experienced physician, my inclination was to provide the remedy without first acknowledging the patient's feelings, struggles, and reaction to the dilemma. I learned. That is not to say that the first word from my mouth has always been "Oy!" But it has been an "oy equivalent," an expression of empathy. A former student told me about this experience in medical school: "While I was accompanying a staff physician, his patient told him of his discomfort from his malignancy and his fears. Though the patient was clearly in distress, the physician listened without reaction. Almost without thinking, I said to the patient, 'This must be very hard for you.' From that moment on in the interview, the patient spoke directly to me and seemed more relaxed."

"The most effective relationships are based on respect, trust and candor."[3] The absence of any one of these three elements undermines the effectiveness of relationships. Honest discussion enhances relationships. Patients want to trust their physician. Even when the news is bad, the physician can be honest about diagnosis, treatment ("These are difficult choices"), prognosis ("Things aren't going well"), psychosocial issues ("You seem depressed; am I reading you right?"), and the relationship itself ("I sense that we're not getting along and I'd like to figure out why").

But patients cannot trust without feeling that they are trusted. It is hard enough to forsake control by entering a hospital or a nursing home; imagine what it must be like if the patient does not trust the doctor, the nurse, or the institution. In turn, the physician should expect complete honesty from the patient. And so every transaction becomes a deposit in a "trust fund." Every transaction is an opportunity either to build or to undermine a trusting relationship. Honesty is one dimension of trust. Some patients have thought it necessary to tell their doctor, "Don't keep anything from me." Left unstated, that worry may linger and attach itself to each transaction. The wise physician says, "I will always be honest with you, for I know that if you ever catch me in a lie, it will be very difficult to reestablish trust."

Start where the patient is. This story, in which the patient's daughter was his surrogate, illustrates how we can get into conflict by ignoring this axiom.

A demented 91-year-old man became tremulous and more breathless at the nursing home. There was no "do not resuscitate" order, and so the patient's nurse called me, and I called his daughter to report the change. Her wishes: Do everything, use a ventilator and resuscitate if necessary. I hospitalized the patient, and because he needed a ventilator to support his breathing, I consulted a pulmonary disease specialist who said he thought the high-technology efforts were a waste of resources for old people, when we live in a community with limited funds.

Whose views should take precedence, the daughter's or the consultant's? What were the issues? Was it cost, prejudice against old people, or paternalism? Was it a difference in the perception of the worth of the old man? For the consultant, the worth had to do with cost to the community. For the daughter, it had to do with her relationship with her father; even though he was demented, he remained an important presence in her life. The daughter and the pulmonary disease specialist saw the dilemma differently.

This interaction was made more difficult because both of us physicians, new to the drama, had no relationship with the daughter, and she needed an ally. We placed her father on a ventilator, and though he died during that hospitalization, the additional time (and money) allowed the daughter to deal with the potential loss. Challenging a point of view without adequate information can undermine the relationship; a far better course is to seek understanding and accommodation. During that time, the physicians and the daughter established an alliance and a shared point of view.

The relationship provides entrée to the medical system. In relation to the entire system of care, the primary physician is the "general contractor" and the patient's advocate. Especially when a complicated illness requires hospitalization and several consultants, the primary doctor becomes the final common pathway for information. Unless one physician is in charge of the message, the patient may get confusing signals from different sources. This story illustrates:

A 60-year-old bachelor had neglected his health for years and was beginning to experience the complications of diabetes, including an infected foot that would not heal. Not one to use fear as a treatment "weapon," I reassured him that with proper treatment and care his foot would heal. My plan, in the long run, was to use this incident and its good outcome as positive reinforcement to alter his style of living. I asked a dietitian to counsel him regarding diet. He repeated to me her exact words: "If you don't take care of yourself, you could lose a foot."

Continuity, knowing the patient over time, is an important dimension. Recall from chapter 1 the patient's requests on the eve of his coronary artery bypass surgery: "Of each of my physicians, cardiologist, and surgeon, I asked for continuity of care—that each would see me daily and be available, rather than a surrogate. I did not want decisions about my care to be made by someone who did not have a complete perspective about me medically. I wanted to be looked after by someone who knew who I was. I did not want too many cooks spoiling the broth. I did not want to feel abandoned."

When I had to tell my 64-year-old patient that his chronic kidney problem had progressed to the point where he now needed dialysis, we were able to have a straightforward conversation. His prior illness had been a long one, and now his wife was seriously ill also. I realized that he and I had a trusting relationship, built up over time, and we could use that relationship in making a difficult decision.

I recognize that patients and families think things over between visits to the doctor, and we ought not necessarily expect an immediate change in an opinion or behavior. If they are not having symptoms, they think about whether or not to have the recommended surgery. They think about the implication of a diagnosis of cancer, heart trouble, or hypertension. At first they may be overwhelmed by the diagnosis, but usually they deal with it in a healthy manner, accept it, and move on to the next step.

Continuity is important, not only for the patient, but also for the physician. When I admitted an 80-year-old woman to the hospital for terminal care, I recognized that this was not simply another hospital admission but also the end of her daughter's long struggle to care for her—a terminal moment for her daughter also. To appreciate the significance of this drama enriched the experience for me and enlarged the opportunities to help each of them. It was important to be able to say to myself, "I *know* you and I can appreciate what you are going through." That comes with continuity and time. Continuity also allows the physician to ruminate about a case, to come up with new insights about the diagnosis and treatment.

Even without the benefits of time, we can develop relationships, especially at moments of great need. I heard this story from a psychiatrist who specialized in caring for patients disabled by industrial accidents.

A young man came to the physician for the first time immediately following an injury to his left wrist. After briefly reviewing the history of the injury, the physician proceeded with his examination. Gently holding his uninjured right arm, he carefully palpated it from elbow to wrist, and declared, "This feels normal." The patient thought, "This doctor at least knows normal from abnormal." Then the doctor examined the injured left arm, starting at the elbow, away from the area of pain. By the time his examining fingers reached the injured, tender wrist, the patient had developed trust in the competence and gentleness of the doctor.

"Think of what it would have been like for the patient," the psychiatrist suggested, "had the physician gone straight for the injured wrist."

This next story is more complex.

A 60-year-old woman saw me for the first time for hypertension, which required medication. After a week, she returned with a more normal blood pressure, but described two brief periods in which she had difficulty speaking. These episodes strongly suggested the diagnosis of a "transient cerebral ischemic attack," related to carotid artery narrowing. Events rapidly unfolded. She had a cerebral angiogram, which showed substantial narrowing of one carotid artery. I referred her to a neurologist who felt, as I did, that the treatment of choice was carotid artery surgery; without it, we felt, she was at risk of a serious stroke. But during the surgery, she had a stroke.

Two challenges arose in this brief relationship, the first one almost immediately. How should I, a doctor new to the woman and her family, present the need for surgery? What I said was, "Here we are, we've hardly met, and I'm already recommending surgery for an illness that's causing you no pain. I recognize how difficult that decision must be for you." Then I went on to explain the details of the difficulty, how the treatment for hypertension had uncovered the previously "silent" (i.e., without symptoms) arterial narrowing, and what the course of her illness might be, treated and untreated. I explored her values. I explained the risks. By doing all of these things, I enhanced my credibility as an involved physician—and not just a technician.

The second challenge was far more difficult. How was I to tell her family that their mother had a stroke during the procedure that was supposed to prevent just such an event? By encouraging her to take this step, we had precipitated this catastrophe. How was I to present this bad news and at the same time deal with their guilt—and mine? First I acknowledged the bad outcome and expressed my sadness. Then I retraced all the steps leading to our decision: the first inkling of the difficulty, the findings on the angiogram, the prognosis of her difficulty with and without treatment, the choices available to us—surgery or medication, and the consensus of all the physicians regarding the best choice. Of the outcome, I said, "You wouldn't be human if you didn't ask, 'Did we, the family, do the right thing?' Like you, I feel badly that this happened. In my mind I retraced all of our steps, and I believe we all made what we thought was the best choice." I also helped the family recognize that the process of dealing with this loss—of good health, speech, and use of one side of her body—takes time.

During the next six months, the patient partially recovered. The relationship, created urgently and quickly, helped get her and her family through this drama. She remained my patient, and other family members became my patients.

The nurse-midwife's creed refers to "being with the patient for as long as it takes." This is another way of saying to a patient, "I will not abandon you." The relationship between the physician and the patient is the key to the human side of medicine.

Chapter 20

What Can Go Wrong with the Doctor-Patient Relationship

"Is this any way to solve a problem?... Is this any way to treat a patient?"

A friend told me the story of a doctor who believed his patient was about to make a decision about his care that would have dangerous consequences and perhaps shorten his life. The patient's decision was based on a number of erroneous assumptions and irrelevant issues. The doctor was getting nowhere in his attempt to redirect the patient's reasoning and finally said to him, "Is this any way to solve a problem?" Sometimes, there is a similar question to ask the doctor: "Is this any way to treat a patient?" Here is what physicians sometimes do that derail the relationship.

Be unavailable. We can be unavailable in many ways, by failing to provide a timely appointment or return phone call or by being physically present but inattentive.

Not care enough to inquire. When a middle-aged woman made many phone calls to her physician in preparation for a breast biopsy, he labeled her "manipulative and demanding" instead of recognizing that she had good reasons for concern and her cascade of questions. She was concerned about how long she would have to be off medication for her chronic illness. In addition, she had a number of prearranged speaking engagements and needed to know which to reschedule. And she was frightened. Her concerns and questions were valid; calling her "manipulative and demanding" was a bum rap.

Stifle the expression of feelings. By interrupting weeping patients, instead of remaining silent and allowing them to show emotion, and by not allowing patients to express anger, fear, anxiety, and doubt, we thereby squander the opportunity to explore these issues and to expand awareness of the patients' stories.

Leave matters unfinished. Physicians leave things unsaid and undone. "After the orthopedist injected my knees with cortisone, both he and his assistant left me. He didn't tell me what I could or couldn't do. There I was, on the examining table. Suppose I couldn't get off the table?" It is not only what we say, but also what we do or do not do.

Lose focus on the patient. Sometimes a family member becomes "the center of the drama." Conflict arises between the physician and the family member because of unrecognized issues. To the detriment of the patient, the family member's issues become paramount. Sometimes physicians become the center of the drama. They feel threatened by a request for another opinion or by questions about their diagnosis or treatment plan. They become defensive when a patient suggests a test that they have not considered. And sometimes the institution becomes the center of the drama. A representative of the hospital or the insurance carrier declares, "The patient no longer needs to be in the hospital" or "This test [consultation, etc.] is not warranted," and the physician accedes prematurely.

Fail to understand that patients have different needs. When a 50-year-old woman called the surgeon's office to ask about the risks of her upcoming spine surgery, the assistant relayed this information from the surgeon to the patient: "You have less than a 5 percent risk of infection, less than a 1 percent risk of paralysis, and less than a 1 percent risk of death." What the patient really needed was a personal conversation with the surgeon to express her fears, get reassurance that the surgery was absolutely necessary, and get his commitment to do all he could to make sure that things turned out well. Not all patients need that comprehensive a response, but it is important that physicians respond to the variability of needs.

Fail to truly grasp what is going on.

Though I generally see my patients at their scheduled time, I was five minutes late for this first meeting with a 75-year-old man who greeted me with, "You're late! Who the hell do you think you are?" Angry and defensive, I was inclined to respond, "I sense that we're not going to get along. I think you should find another doctor." Instead I asked myself, "What's his anger all about? What's *my* anger all about?" I recognized that he reminded me of someone who had been depressed for many years; *his* anger was an expression of his depression. Instead of dismissing the patient, who was indeed depressed, I relaxed, continued the interview, and used that insight in his care.

In this mental exercise, which took less than thirty seconds, I applied what I had been taught in medical school: Part of the mental status examination of a patient, is asking yourself the question, "What's my reaction to the patient and what does my reaction mean?"

Not recognize where the patient is in the story. When a patient has been dealing with another illness, physician, and set of assumptions for a long time, it is no wonder that she may initially reject a new physician's opinions.

Expect patients to make decisions too quickly. Difficult decisions cannot be made in a moment.

Patients' and families' behavior, too, can have a negative impact on relationships with physicians. Here are two common ways.

Misinterpret the physician's motives. When the son of a nursing home resident called to request psychiatric consultation for his mother who had become confused, I suggested an alternative: "I'll see her first to look for nonpsychiatric causes of her confusion." He rejected the proposal, accusing me of "trying to save the state some money by being 'the gatekeeper.'" A relationship would have helped. The son had clearly constructed his own story about me.

Sometimes it is appropriate and necessary to confront a patient about inappropriate behavior, an opportunity to discover previously unidentified issues and strengthen the relationship. "Very few people can be cured by a doctor they do not like. . . . [As a doctor], I have never been able to do much for a patient I thoroughly disliked."[1] If the relationship is consistently adversarial, the physician needs to ask, "Why? What are the issues?" and sometimes, that it is a reason to recommend that the patient find another doctor.

Continually shop around for another physician. Lacking trust and an ongoing relationship, patients may wander from doctor to doctor and self-refer to specialists who do not have the whole story.

The worst of what can go wrong? *Neither the patient nor the physician expects a relationship, and neither realizes what is missing.*

THE DIFFICULT PATIENT

One of the largest groups of patients whose needs go unmet are the so-called "difficult patients." Often these patients have one or more of these characteristics:

An elusive diagnosis. Despite persistence of his symptoms over a period of weeks or months, his health is not deteriorating. Tests for various common and rarely occurring illnesses are normal, even when done repeatedly. The story does not fit the pattern of any known disease. His chest pain is unrelated to a disease of the heart, lungs, or other chest contents; his abdominal pain has no obvious source in any of the abdominal organs. His illness contrasts starkly with that of the patient whose symptoms persist, whose health is failing, who is obviously ill, and yet the physicians cannot yet determine the cause. We have all heard examples: the patient with unexplained chest pain who, after many months and extensive medical consultation, has a severe heart attack; the patient with unexplained abdominal pain who ultimately is diagnosed with cancer of the ovary or pancreas, illnesses that may be difficult to detect in their early stages. The physicians know something is wrong, but no one can come up with the answer.

An inappropriately prolonged recovery. Despite an illness that has been adequately diagnosed and treated, the patient is not *feeling* better. All the parameters indicating successful treatment are improving, yet the patient feels the same or worse.

Difficult rapport. Even though all the elements of a good doctor-patient relationship are present, the patient distrusts the physician and the relationship is—well—difficult.

Like the butcher with persistent back pain (chapter 9), the "difficult patient" is often dealing with important psychological or social issues. Identifying these issues and providing integrated and thoughtful continuity of care can be transformative. Suddenly a relationship develops, and the diagnostic and therapeutic questions resolve.

But we cannot take these steps in the care of the patient without this insight: Just as the problem "congestive heart failure" (Table 20.1) has a list of symptoms that, taken alone or together, suggest a differential diagnosis, so does the problem "difficult patient" (Table 20.2). Just as we may name the problem "congestive heart failure" on the basis of one or more of symptoms, so we would make the problem statement "difficult patient" on the basis of one or more criteria.

Difficult patients with elusive diagnoses may have a real, though not obvious, disease; just as likely, the illness may be related to psychosocial problems. A difficult patient who is not feeling better despite adequate treatment may lack progress not because of an undetected complication, but because of distressing life events. When there is no rapport, despite the physician's best efforts, the cause may be psychosocial.

As part of the differential diagnosis of "difficult patient," I included in Table 20.2 "difficult doctor" and "difficult system," a view parallel to those

Table 20.1
Congestive Heart Failure: Symptoms and Differential Diagnosis

- Symptoms: shortness of breath, poor exercise tolerance, rapid heartbeat, ankle swelling
- Differential diagnosis: coronary heart disease, valvular heart disease, primary disease of the heart muscle (cardiomyopathy)

Table 20.2
"Difficult Patient": Symptoms and Differential Diagnosis

- Symptoms: Diagnosis is elusive, recovery is prolonged, rapport between patient and physician is difficult to establish
- Differential diagnosis: organic disease, e.g., difficult-to-diagnose malignancy, unusual cause of chest or abdominal pain, other rarely occurring disease; psychosocial problems; "difficult doctor"; "difficult system"

in the book entitled *There Are No Problem Horses, Only Problem Riders*.[2] If the physician consistently deals with each patient with equanimity, then how the patient behaves can be seen as possible data on how the patient deals with others. If, on the other hand, the physician is inconsistent and uneven—if the patient cannot trust that the doctor will be the same on each encounter or if the physician's demeanor is provocative—then how the patient behaves cannot be seen as data. The doctor will always have to ask, "Was it the patient who provoked this response or was it me?" Or additionally, "Did the system contribute to making this patient difficult, by not meeting his needs?"

A colleague suggested that "any difficult patient started out as a complex patient." Patients whose illnesses are complex or who have complex dramas going on in their lives may have difficulty in finding a physician with enough patience to address all the issues. Incomplete attention may leave the patient dissatisfied and frustrated. When that happens, the physician also becomes frustrated, labels the patient "difficult," the prophesy is self-fulfilled, and no one feels satisfied. But not all complex patients become difficult, and not all difficult patients are that complex in the right hands. Just as physicians see serious illnesses as a challenge, many physicians see "difficult patients" as challenges also. The search for the solutions to these challenges becomes fascinating, and their resolution elevates everyone. Anyone can deal with easy problems or patients. One test of good doctors—real professionals—is how they deal with the difficult ones.

Social workers learn this axiom: "The relationship is the vehicle." Like any relationship, that between doctor and patient can be used well or abused. Once trust is established, it can be a model for other relationships. Robert Coles writes about what his teacher taught him about dealing with a difficult patient: "Try to learn, and if she can use you to her advantage [and] profit from the relationship and the insight you offer, well and good."[3] If the relationship is a good one, it can be a model to the patient for other relationships. A good relationship facilitates diagnosis, treatment, and overall care.

Chapter 21

Addressing Some of the Myths about the Doctor-Patient Relationship

"How can I keep from becoming emotionally involved?"

In a class for first-year medical students, excerpts from Anatole Broyard's book, *Intoxicated by My Illness*, are required reading. In it, Broyard, faced with the diagnosis of prostate cancer, declared his requirements for a physician: "not only a talented physician, but a bit of a metaphysician, too. Someone who can treat body and soul . . . [one] who *enjoyed* me."[1] In response to the reading, a student asked me, "How can I keep from becoming emotionally involved?"[2] The question had additional weight because several of her classmates in the section had responded to my question, "What is the most important issue facing you now as a physician-in-training?" with these answers: "becoming too emotionally involved" and "losing my humanity." Patients and friends had often asked me the same question. And Robert Coles took note of this issue when he wrote in *The Call of Stories*, "I learned [from my teaching supervisor] that it was best for me not to get 'too involved.'"[3]

The class discussion made it clear that the students saw "emotionally involved" as a pejorative term. It implied weakness on the part of the physician. It implied that we would become less effective and less professional and would lose our objectivity. It was dangerous to become emotionally involved, placing ourselves at risk of having our practice "take over" our personal life.

In fact, good physicians do their job in a sensitive, involved way and avoid these pitfalls. And so I believe that seeing the term "emotionally involved" in a negative way is invalid. Centering the discussion around the question as the student asked it would have tainted and inappropriately confined the discussion. I thought that we should reframe the question before we proceeded, and so I proposed this continuum: At one end was "cold," as in "That doctor is a 'cold fish.'" At the other end was "emotionally involved." And in the middle was, well, "the middle."

cold————the middle————emotionally involved

We agreed that either extreme was undesirable.

I asked the students to define the middle. They answered: "Finding out what it's like for patients, taking time with them, going beyond the technical aspects of their illness. Understanding that an illness may have impact on patients' income, the viability of their career, and on their self-image. Finding out what it's like for families. Recognizing that illness is a family experience. Understanding that an illness may have impact on the dynamics of family life. Asking the appropriate questions to address those issues." They recognized already that developing a sense of the patient's experience through interested inquiry could not only enhance the relationship between the patient, the family, and the physician but also might affect the process of care and even improve the outcome.

To their definition of "the middle," they added: "Empathy and understanding. Not simply an awareness of what it's like, but an expression to the patient of that understanding. Saying it!" Sad to say, many patients no longer expect that from their physicians. "Saying it" signals the patient that the physician is "involved," may have thought about the patient's experience, perhaps even wondered, "What would it be like if it were me?" and has thought about issues beyond the technical ones.

"Sitting at the bedside rather than standing," one student offered. We had talked previously about patients' perception that a seated hospital visit *seemed* longer than a standing one. They recognized that not only was it acceptable, it was *advisable* to involve oneself in an inquiry about what it was like for the patient, but also to do it in a way that seemed unhurried to the patient. Sitting meant that the physician was not in a hurry, that the patient at that moment had her undivided attention. Patients often note other body language and subtle signs of interest and involvement: eye contact, concentration on what the patient was saying, validation of what was said with restatements and further inquiry, and expressing respect for the patient's point of view and values. They also noticed when these qualities were absent in their physicians. The "middle," then, is a continuum. There are many appropriate, yet not excessive, aspects of involvement.

"What is excessive involvement?" I then asked the students. "What is 'too involved'? What breaches the threshold between 'the middle' and 'emotionally involved'?" "Babysitting for the patient's children" was one answer. I followed up by asking, "What are 'babysitting' equivalents?" Providing care at a discounted fee is appropriate; paying patients' rent bills or loaning them money is inappropriate. Participating in a prayer with a patient at his request is appropriate; initiating prayer is not, for it may be improperly imposing the physician's values upon the patient. Intent is important. Touching with romantic intent is inappropriate; touching to comfort is not. At the edge, of course, was sexual involvement or meeting a patient for a drink.

"Doctors' inappropriate sharing of their personal lives" was another answer. It may be acceptable for doctors to comment on their own experience of illness in order to validate for the patient that they understand the patient's struggles. On the other hand, it would be inappropriate for physicians to discuss their own family conflicts and financial dilemmas. "Allowing ourselves to take on the patient's burdens. Not seeing that we are going beyond our skills."

"Could someone be an effective physician for a relative or friend?" Addressing this question seemed to complement the larger discussion and further clarify the issue. Practicing in a small community—a small town or ethnic community—we can hardly avoid taking care of friends and relatives. And it works. The lesson for all care is clear: So long as doctors do not inappropriately taint their decisions or alter basic patterns of diagnosis, treatment, and interaction, they avoid the dangers of becoming "emotionally involved."

We explored the meaning of "cold," at the other end of the spectrum: "The physician doesn't talk at all, doesn't connect at all. The physician sees only the technical aspects of the medical problem."

When we completed the discussion, we renamed the entire continuum of involvement. Just as we realized that "emotionally involved" was a phrase burdened with too many negative connotations, we also realized that "cold" was pejorative. We changed the continuum from:

cold———the middle———emotionally involved

to

uninvolved———involved———inappropriately involved

Doing so allowed us latitude to consider the dimensions of involvement without being defensive. It allowed us to say that involvement is a virtue of being a good doctor or, better yet, a requirement. This story from my practice illustrates.

In his mid-60s, a retired laboratory technician had most of the complications of diabetes mellitus: His vision was failing, the circulation to his legs was impaired, nerve injury hampered his ability to feel pain in his feet, and his heart muscle, injured by previous heart attacks, pumped inefficiently. Now he was hospitalized for the third time in as many months for kidney failure, with fluid accumulated in his lungs and an accompanying disorder of body chemistry. While renal dialysis was an option, it was clearly only a short-term solution, one of many that seemed to divert him and his wife from dealing with his approaching death.

Here were my options for involvement:

- Uninvolved: Simply addressing the urgent technical issues—treating the congestive heart failure and the kidney failure with medication and dialysis and treating the diabetes with insulin.
- Inappropriately involved: Taking his and his wife's burden as my own; taking their anticipated loss as my own.
- Involved: My concern was that they not squander this precious and uncertain time in futile therapeutic maneuvers and false hopes. I was concerned also that when the patient died, his wife not be faced with a grief prolonged by the feelings that "if only he and I had talked more, if only I had said once more how much our relationship meant," and "I wonder if I did all I could." I wanted to help provide them with the time to deal with concrete matters, legal and otherwise, and emotional matters.

I chose to be involved. The patient, his wife, and I addressed these issues together and agreed to cease vigorous treatment beyond that related to his comfort. The patient died a week later. In a letter after his death, his wife thanked me for "the precious week that [he] and I had." What I had done was not trivial.

Physicians and others have taken the position that involvement, described this way, is more properly the role of someone else—social workers, nurses, clergy, psychologists. Besides, "It takes too much time, and physicians' time is better spent in other activities that only they can do." But who else is in a better position to do it than the physician? Our knowledge of the patient, details and nuances of the illness, its uncertainties and prognosis, our ongoing *presence* and our *relationship* with the patient and the family make us uniquely qualified to participate in the patient's care in this way.

What about the concern that being involved takes too much time? My conversation with this couple, enabling them to explore these important issues, took a few minutes. Each prior transaction through the years of his illness was a deposit in the "trust account" of our relationship; our long relationship validated the current series of transactions. It simply does not take much time to do this.

Another concern, and perhaps the real concern, is that the accumulation of every involved transaction will ultimately overwhelm the physician. If involvement is seen as appropriate and *necessary*, in the same way that taking a thorough medical history and doing a physical examination are, and if it is seen as a continuum, done more or less as the circumstances require, then it will not be overwhelming. On the contrary, it will be measured, appropriate, and satisfying.

Both patients and physicians need the reinforcement and validation of the relationship. I recall a moment in the fall of 1998, when two women who had breast cancer spoke to the first-year medical school class at the University of Minnesota about their reactions to the illness and its impact on their lives. During the question-and-answer period, two students rose to thank them and then the entire class gave them a standing ovation, both extraordinary responses to a medical lecture. By so doing, they validated them as patients and as their teachers. In effect they said: "We heard what you said. We understand—or can begin to understand—what it has been like for you. We admire the way you've handled things and have a great deal of respect for you."

One may think that these women did not need that. After all, they had long since demonstrated their strength by coming so far. But all of us—patients, students, teachers, and physicians—need validation, and it does not have to be in the form of a standing ovation. It can be something as simple as saying, "That's some story. I can only begin to imagine what this must have been like for you. You deserve a lot of credit for the way you've handled things." Given a choice, a moment's pause about whether or not to do it, just do it. It is another way to be involved.

What does the "involvement," the relationship, mean? For the patient, the physician's involvement dignifies the transaction by taking it beyond a technical exercise to one of humanity and caring. It allows the patient to reflect, "This doctor I'm dealing with is a complete person. She understands. She understands *me*. In the matter of my illness, we are equal partners." Especially when the illness is complex, involvement provides reassurance that the patient has an advocate, a "general contractor," someone who knows what questions to ask, who provides the authorization to have feelings and fears, and who can help address those feelings. Involvement enriches all the transactions. Absent involvement, the patient and the family miss support at the very least, but also they can miss the opportunity to explore options, uncertainty, and values and to plan thoughtfully for the future.

But the relationship works both ways. For the physician, it is affirming and enriching. An undergraduate wrote, "The human experience is one of great depth and wisdom and I am continually amazed at the strength and resilience we seem to show time and time again. As a physician, I would be able to witness these wonders of the human spirit, and in this way I feel it would be a great honor to be a healer." It is reinforcing to have an appreciative, long-standing patient. When the relationship makes the patient feel better, it makes the doctor feel better. Lacking involvement sterilizes the transaction. Without involvement, each patient with abdominal pain becomes just one more case rather than an opportunity for exploration and discovering new insights about people and their lives. Broyard again: "It doesn't take much time to make good contact, but beyond that, the emotional burden of *avoiding* the patient may be much harder on the doctor than he imagines."[4] And author Anne Lamott describes a conversation with her dying friend's doctor: " 'Watch her carefully right now,' she said, 'because she's teaching you how to live.' "[5]

"People fulfill themselves as human beings through relationships," my friends were charged during their wedding ceremony. Absent the relationship, both patient and physician lose.

PART IV

THE HUMAN SIDE OF MEDICINE: BRINGING IT ALL TOGETHER

Chapter 22

Another Look at a Day in the Life of a Physician

"Routines, routines, routines."

This chapter reprises chapter 8, "A Day in the Life of a Physician." Now I show how to use the book's lessons with most of the patients from that chapter. Exploring the patient's *story* enhances the validity of the *history* and helps to define the *issues*. The *doctor-patient relationship* facilitates the whole process. Asking *"What did I learn?"* in the office, at the patient's home, or the hospital bedside turns each encounter into a moment of enhanced care and professional growth.

Besides the intellectual challenge and the opportunity to serve, this routine keeps the physician stimulated and fulfilled. Good, careful, thorough physicians do all of this naturally. The time that it takes is crucial to good care. For patients, the consistent exercise of such a routine validates the physician's commitment to them; they see it in the ways the doctor talks and takes action.

In the long term, such care depends on a good medical record. Together, the "five steps," the problem-oriented record, and the biopsychosocial model provide useful and reproducible frameworks for practice. The medical record becomes a compendium of the physician's insights, how our mind was working at the time we made a complex decision, and what works and what does not. Alone and together with records of other patients, it is a resource for self-teaching. A day's worth of patients provides a year's worth of lessons.

As I reprise the day, the dimensions of the human side of medicine stand out. I use the convention of preceding each with the symbol **H**.

THE HOSPITAL

Hospital patients tend to be complex and have many ongoing problems rather than a single one. They often have many physicians and other health professionals involved in their care.

(Refer to the corresponding cases in chapter 8. Refer also to the commentaries in that chapter for an explanation of unfamiliar technical terms.)

Patient 1: A.B., Age 29

The Physician's Note in the Chart

Abdominal pain and weight loss: Still no appetite. Tests, including proctoscopy, barium enema, endoscopy of stomach, and CT scan of abdomen, show a small ovarian mass. Thyroid tests are normal.

Seizures: now and then.

Her abdominal pain and weight loss are very likely multidetermined—related to her antiseizure medication and the psychosocial issues in her life. Prior to discharge, we need to settle the medication issue and arrange for adequate psychiatric follow-up.

Additional Story, Additional History

For years she has had seizures, not well controlled despite use of various medications, and there is some question as to whether or not she is taking the medicines in the prescribed dose. During the last few months, she has lost 20 pounds, and has had some unexplained abdominal pain. Her life is in disarray. She has recently become engaged, and her fiancé is making unreasonable sexual demands. She can no longer afford her apartment. She has no family or friends she can consistently turn to for moral support. Her medical care has become divided among a neurologist, an internist, a psychiatrist, a psychiatric social worker, and a social worker from the welfare department, and she does not know who is in charge.

The Issues

- What is the cause of her weight loss? Does she have a malignancy or an overactive thyroid gland? Are her medications for seizures causing her to lose weight? H Is what is going on in her life contributing to her weight loss?

- Does the ovarian mass discovered on her CT scan require further investigation to rule out an endocrine disorder or malignancy, or is it an incidental finding of no consequence?

- H Who is in charge of her care—the neurologist looking after her seizures, the internist, the psychiatrist who has seen her previously and referred her to a day care program, or the patient herself? Is part of her illness related to her sense of panic that, in the face of her own inadequate system of support, no one seems to be overseeing her care?

The Doctor-Patient Relationship

- I reassure her that she has no malignancy.

- H I arrange for the neurologist to coordinate her care, to manage her seizure medications, and to be certain that she is getting adequate psychiatric follow-up.

- H I call her to summarize these plans, and I arrange to see her in two weeks. I tell her that I am available, even though I am not her primary physician.

What Did I Learn?

- Some decisions are complex.

- Single problems (abdominal pain, weight loss, loss of appetite) can be multidetermined.

- H Weight loss has many causes, including organic ones and those having a psychological and social basis.

- Resolution of some problems takes time.

- H Psychosocial issues may intrude upon a physical illness and prevent its timely resolution.

- H Patients may panic when their medical care is so divided among various professionals that no one seems to be in charge. One person needs to coordinate care and present a consistent message.

Patient 2: C.D., Age 85.

The Note

Back pain: persists. X-ray shows osteoporosis of the lumbar spine and old compression fractures but no new ones. Her exam is unchanged. She rarely requires pain medication.

Additional Story, Additional History

Despite her failing memory over the last several years, she has managed to remain at home with help from a home-delivered meal program, periodic visits from a homemaker, and phone calls and visits from her brothers. Bladder cancer has been treated with chemotherapy. She also has aortic insufficiency, a heart valve defect. The recent onset of back pain has pushed her over the threshold of self-sufficiency; she can no longer get around or be alone.

The Issues

- Has tumor spread caused her back pain? Are there other possible causes of her back pain?

- **H** Where should she live? At home with live-in help or in a nursing home? The main dilemma is not her back pain, for acute fracture and tumor have been ruled out and pain is easily controlled by oral medication. But she is vulnerable and can no longer be alone.

The Doctor-Patient Relationship

- **H** I recognize that she cannot be responsible for important decisions in her care because of her failing memory and impaired judgment. I define the issues for her brother, who is acting in her behalf.

- **H** I recognize that the transition from home to a nursing home is a difficult and delicate one. I help provide her with not only a safe place but also enough time for thoughtful and adequate planning. I also provide moral support for the brother who feels guilty about moving her to the nursing home. "You've done all you possibly could for her," I tell him. I involve the hospital social worker in these plans, and I assure the brother that he need not fear that his sister will be discharged from the hospital prematurely.

What Did I Learn?

- Back pain has a number of possible causes, each of which has a different remedy.

- **H** Part of the assessment of any patient is inquiring about what is going on in her life. For this patient, addressing *only* the issue of the back pain would not have solved her problem.

- **H** The role of the physician is not only to provide diagnostic and therapeutic support to the patient and her family but also moral and emotional support.

Patient 3: E.F., Age 85

The Note

Fever and lightheadedness: She's no longer lightheaded. Fever has disappeared.

Potassium deficit: has been corrected.

Additional Story, Additional History

Unlike Patient C.D., who is exactly the same age, this lady has a sharp mind, is independent, lives alone, and conducts a very active life. What brought her to the hospital was an acute episode of dizziness associated with fever. For years she has had hypertension, treated with hydrochlorothiazide and a potassium supplement. Her hospitalization is a brief one, and while all the issues are not settled by the time of her hospital discharge, I feel that she and I can resolve them after she returns home.

The Issues

- What is the cause of her fever? Does she have pneumonia, a bladder infection, the "flu," or some other less obvious cause? Is she sufficiently ill to require an immediate extensive evaluation of the fever, or can I delay tests for a day or two and make further observations only if she gets worse?

- What is the cause of her dizziness—dehydration, fever, the blood pressure drug, or all three? Is her illness multidetermined?

- The blood potassium concentration is low. Is she taking her medication correctly?

The Doctor-Patient Relationship

- H Because I have been her physician for ten years, she knows that she can call me at any time if she feels worse and I know that she is sufficiently reliable to follow up as I have suggested. We are both comfortable with her returning home before all the issues are settled.

What Did I Learn?

- The presence of a problem, such as fever, may not require an immediate extensive evaluation.

- H Age alone does not define how vigorous and self-sufficient a person is.

- H Knowing a patient over a long period of time provides valuable insights for making difficult decisions.

Patient 4: G.H., Age 78

The Note

Fever: improving. No cough, no chills. Urinalysis is normal. Chest x-ray normal.

Diabetes mellitus: Blood sugars are in the 100–200 range on a mixture of NPH and regular insulin.

Coronary heart disease: no breathlessness, no chest pain, no significant arrhythmia.

Thought disorder: He is still combative, and he won't talk to me.

Exam: Alert, does not look acutely ill. Chest: clear. Heart: regular rhythm.

Etiology of the fever is still unclear, though he is improving on intravenous antibiotic.

Additional Story, Additional History

This elderly man recently emigrated from the Soviet Union. In the last few months, he has been faced with an avalanche of illnesses, starting with complete heart block (a cardiac conduction disturbance), with associated congestive heart failure and respiratory failure, which required insertion of a cardiac pacemaker and use of a ventilator. Then he developed phlebitis in his leg, requiring anticoagulation. He has diabetes mellitus requiring insulin. In the nursing home, he had become suspicious of his physician and his nurses, ultimately refusing all of his medications. Hampered by the language barrier, a psychiatrist was unable to help decide if he was depressed, delusional, or confused. His new problem, unexplained fever, is superimposed upon all these other problems. His responsible family member, a daughter, is bewildered by the complexity of his illness and its related problems.

The Issues

- What is the cause of his fever? Does he have pneumonia, an infection in his urinary tract, or a pulmonary embolus (a blood clot in his lungs)?

- What therapeutic decisions need to be made for the diabetes mellitus, the coronary heart disease, and the fever of unknown origin? In the face of these uncertainties, can I begin treatment without knowing the definite diagnosis?

- What is the cause of his combativeness? Of all the causes, some are not treatable. Which ones are?

- H What compromises need to be made regarding ideal management for this "difficult" patient? What does it mean to be a difficult patient?

- **H** Does the daughter or anyone else in the family need attention from the physician?

The Doctor-Patient Relationship

- **H** Faced with an uncooperative patient who is at high risk for progression of his illness, I alert the family members, recognize their own struggle, and help them make responsible decisions in their father's behalf.

What Did I Learn?

- I add to my practical list of possible causes of fever.

- Beyond the technical tasks of managing each of this patient's illnesses, named and yet to be named, is recognizing that his combativeness is itself a problem that needs to be more clearly defined.

- Not every problem has a solution.

Patient 5: I.J., Age 68

The Note

Congestive heart failure: Overall he feels much better. Not breathless. Slept well. He has lost 10 pounds since admission, on varying doses of furosemide.

Exam: Pulse 60, irregular. Blood pressure 120/80. He weeps as he speaks of his illnesses. Neck veins flat at 30 degrees. Chest: clear. Heart: irregular rhythm, variable S-1 as before. Liver: not palpable. No presacral or pretibial edema.

Gout: Erythema and pain in his hand have resolved.

Pelvic tumor: no symptoms.

Additional Story, Additional History

He has been hospitalized because of a recurrence of congestive heart failure, which began when he started taking indomethacin for an acute episode of gout and, on his own, had stopped taking a diuretic drug. Fifteen years previously, a rare type of pelvic cancer had been removed, and he had declined follow-up examinations. Eighteen months ago, the tumor recurred and required partial bladder resection. Around that time, he had his first episode of congestive heart failure and a cardiac rhythm disturbance called atrial fibrillation. The electrocardiogram showed a myocardial infarct, though he could not recall any moment of severe chest pain. Again he declined medical follow-up and any tests to determine the state of his tumor.

The Issues

- What is the cause of his congestive heart failure? Could any of the drug changes have precipitated the episode of congestive heart failure?
- In the face of atrial fibrillation and congestive heart failure, is he at extra risk for blood clot formation? Does he need preventive treatment with anticoagulation medicine? Is the presence of tumor a contraindication to the use of anticoagulation medicine?
- What is the best management for his rare tumor—chemotherapy, irradiation, a combination of the two, or nothing at all? His tumor is so rare that there are insufficient data to support preference for any of these choices to answer this question.
- **H** Why does he weep? Is he depressed? What are his fears? How does he interpret his condition?
- **H** What ethical issues are raised if he declines recommended treatment?
- **H** How does the physician integrate the patient's values into making a decision about therapy?

The Doctor-Patient Relationship

- **H** I explore his understanding of his illness and his feelings. I ask, "What's this like for you?"

What Did I Learn?

- Certain diagnoses, such as congestive heart failure, need to be further defined as to cause, for the treatment may depend on the cause.
- Much illness is drug or treatment induced. When a new medicine or treatment is prescribed or stopped, we need to anticipate all the possible effects of the change. Indomethacin can precipitate congestive heart failure.
- Certain tumors and other illnesses may have a tendency to bleed, and so they preclude use of anticoagulant drugs. Certain problems may preclude certain treatment of other problems. To be especially safe, physicians need to examine the interactions between problems and treatments.
- **H** There is uncertainty in medicine. Sometimes the answers to difficult questions, such as the prognosis and treatment of rare tumors, may yet be unavailable.
- **H** Physicians need to integrate the patient's values into decisions.
- **H** Hospitalized or not, a competent patient has the right to refuse care.

THE OFFICE

Office patients can have single, simple problems. Just as often, they may have multiple, complex ones, though they are generally not as acutely ill as hospitalized patients. The first two cases, "annual physicals," are an opportunity to review the year and attend to all the medical and psychosocial issues in depth. Each of these encounters lasts forty-five to sixty minutes.

Patient 6: K.L., Age 45

The Note

A 45-year-old woman here for annual physical. Problems are as follows:

Myxomatous mitral valve, post mitral valve replacement: on warfarin. No chest pain. No breathlessness. No awareness of irregular heartbeat. EKG today shows sinus bradycardia, rate about 56, with frequent ventricular extrasystoles and first-degree a-v block.

Thought disorder: ongoing.

Weight loss: a new problem. Weight 14 months ago was 150 and now is 138. She says she is struggling financially and often does not eat well. No special weather preference to suggest hyperthyroidism.

Medications: warfarin and some over-the-counter health-food preparations.

Review of systems is otherwise essentially negative.

Psychosocial: Though she is struggling financially, she does not consistently turn to anyone for moral support. She knows that she can rely on her niece.

Impression: Weight loss, probably due to inadequate nutrition. Urged to eat better.

Arrhythmia, as noted above. Probably not clinically significant.

With her permission, I will speak with her niece.

Return in 3 months.

Additional Story, Additional History

For many years, she had an abnormal heart valve, at first without symptoms and then aggravated by an attacker's stab wound to the chest, which required emergency open-heart surgery. She later developed congestive heart failure and required a second heart surgery for insertion of an artificial mitral valve. Within a year, she developed endocarditis, a serious infection of the artificial valve, after a minor dental procedure. Her cardiac status is now stable. She takes warfarin to prevent blood clot formation around the valve.

Though she has a long-standing thought disorder, she is college educated, and with her technical background, she has had steady employment, though now it is sporadic. Because of the psychiatric disorder, she is more vulnerable: She has made some unwise financial decisions that now partially explain her current financial bind. She has no living parents or siblings, though she relies on her niece and knows she could turn to her in an emergency.

The Issues

- Is her cardiac status stable and satisfactory?
- Is it a coincidence that the episode of endocarditis followed the minor dental procedure? Are there measures to prevent recurrence?
- What is the cause of her weight loss? H Is it related to poor nutrition, and if so, is this a consequence of her unwise financial decisions and inadequate income?
- H Is she able to make sound judgments? Is she a vulnerable adult? Do family members need to be involved? What are the ethical issues?

The Doctor-Patient Relationship

- H My long-term relationship with the patient allows me to discuss some very personal questions: What are her financial resources? To whom can she turn for moral and financial support? Respecting her privacy, I ask her for permission to talk with her niece about her health and the financial issues.

What Did I Learn?

- Though not all events are caused by preceding ones, the episode of endocarditis may have been caused by the dental work. For future dental procedures, she should take prophylactic antibiotic treatment.
- H Ethical issues occur frequently in the course of medical practice.

Patient 7: M.N., Age 50

The Note

A 50-year-old woman here for annual physical. Problems are as follows:

Diabetes mellitus: no weakness, numbness, or tingling of face, arms, or legs, nausea, diarrhea, change in vision. She has periodic eye checkups by ophthalmologist and retinologist. No symptoms to suggest hypoglycemia. She is on this insulin regimen: regular insulin 12 to 18 units before breakfast, lunch, and supper, and NPH 30 units before supper. She does not regularly test her blood sugar but chooses the amount of insulin according to how active she is going to be. She has given up sweets and finds that there are fewer swings in her blood sugar when she does test.

Hypertension: no headaches or dizziness. On Vasotec, 5 mg daily.

Asthma: rare wheezing. She takes albuterol, 2 puffs, before she runs and as needed, and Theodur, 600 mg twice a day.

Caffeine excess: drinks about two cups of coffee a day and one or two cans of caffeinated cola a day.

Possible allergy to penicillin.

Ethanol, nicotine, and drug excess: none for many years.

Rectal bleeding: none.

Epigastric burning: none

Impaired hearing: unchanged.

Review of systems is otherwise essentially negative.

Psychosocial: All in all, things are going well for her. She has taken on new work responsibilities, shares her feelings with her husband. She was offered a job in another city, the equivalent of a promotion, but chose to remain here.

Impression: Diabetes mellitus: adequate control for her. Check Hgb A1C.

Hypertension: adequately controlled.

Asthma: adequately controlled.

Plan: Continue current regimen. Call me in 4 days for test results and further discussion.

Additional Story, Additional History

She developed diabetes as a teenager, at which time I became her physician. In the course of time, she admitted to abusing drugs and alcohol, and she also smoked. For many years, she struggled with these addictions and the associated disruptions in her life, while also having to deal with the regimentation of the diabetes treatment. Ultimately she conquered all of her addictions, has a successful and fulfilling career working in drug rehabilitation, and a good, honest, and open marriage. The management of her diabetes has been a compromise, which she and I have recognized, periodically revalidated, and renegotiated. Over the years, she has become more and more attentive to her diabetic care.

The Issues

- **H** Beyond the named illnesses—diabetes mellitus, asthma, and hypertension—I need to attend to habits that may adversely affect the patient's health, including nicotine, caffeine, alcohol, and drug consumption.

The Doctor-Patient Relationship

- **H** I need to manage the diabetes in the context of what is going on in her life, know when to compromise, and be sufficiently honest enough to acknowledge the compromise. A straightforward and open relationship facilitates such discussions and also becomes a model to the patient for dealing with other dilemmas in her life. While the control of her blood sugar level is not ideal, she is unable to discipline herself further, and I cannot ignore the other successes she has had in overcoming her addictions.

What Did I Learn?

- **H** Sometimes important information, especially that of a sensitive nature such as substance abuse, may not be obtained on the first interview. The physician must always be open to readdressing the patient's story.

- **H** The story is never over. Her chaotic life, disrupted by addiction and diabetes, evolved into an ordered and productive one, with fulfilling relationships.

- **H** That a person has diabetes mellitus ("is a diabetic") does not define her. As physicians, we often define a person too narrowly and explain away all disruptions with the diagnosis of a chronic illness such as diabetes. ("Who wouldn't be upset, angry, depressed, etc., if they had diabetes?") Such a narrow view limits fruitful inquiry.

- **H** In caring for patients and managing illness, we often compromise the ideal to fit with the individual patient's life and capability for adjustment. Both the physician and the patient need to recognize the compromises and renegotiate them from time to time.

The next series of transactions include shorter office visits, up to fifteen minutes, and telephone calls usually not exceeding five minutes. Even these briefer transactions have human dimensions. Throughout the day, the office staff and I exchange information and instructions.

Patient 8: I.J., Age 68 (Telephone—Son)

The Note

We talked about some of the issues involved in his father's hospitalization (congestive heart failure, underlying heart disease, unusual tumor) and some of the uncertainties related to the illness.

Additional Story, Additional History

The caller is the son of Patient 5, I.J., who is currently hospitalized.

The Issues

- **H** What are the best posthospital plans?

The Doctor-Patient Relationship

- **H** The involved family helps to look after this man's best interests. They are also suffering. My role is to help them with information, guidance in making posthospital arrangements, and moral support. At the same time, the family provides me with valuable information regarding the patient's resources, and they help to validate decisions related to plans following discharge.

What Did I Learn?

- **H** Illness is a family affair. Each family member has needs and can be a valuable source of information and an important part of the collaborative team.

Patient 9: O.P., Age 72 (Telephone)

The Note

Goiter: Repeat TSH is low. I spoke with my colleague, Dr. S, and also with Dr. M, the radiation therapist, about further evaluation and treatment. The nodule is "cold" on the 1989 radioactive scan, but thyroid aspiration was normal. To repeat the scan now to look for any changes. Further decisions about treatment will be made after the scan.

Additional Story, Additional History

The patient is a widow, and so she has to deal with each new crisis alone. She has had a prior encounter with malignancy, cancer of the breast, for which she had a radical mastectomy many years ago, and so she has dealt with many of the issues of malignancy: uncertainty, loss, and the possibility of premature death. She has also dealt successfully with depression.

The Issues

- Is the goiter, a swelling of the usually small thyroid gland, a sign of malignancy? What is the best way to tell, short of surgical removal of the thyroid gland? Does the long-standing presence of the enlargement, unchanged over the years, absolutely rule out the presence of the malignancy? If malignancy is present, what is the best treatment for it?
- **H** How will she handle the news of a possible new malignancy?

The Doctor-Patient Relationship

- **H** I have been her physician for many years, and so I can raise the question of malignancy and offer her credible information and realistic reassurance. Even if the goiter is malignant and she requires consultation and treatment from a surgeon and others, she knows that I will shepherd her through this new crisis, offering her advice and support along the way.

What Did I Learn?

- The long-standing presence of a goiter may hide subtle subsequent changes of malignancy. (I had learned this when caring for another patient.)
- Medicine is a collaborative profession. I consulted with an endocrinologist and a radiation therapist regarding her thyroid.
- H We need not be reluctant to present potentially bad news.

Patient 10: Q.R., Age 78 (Telephone)

The Note

Tongue biopsy was negative for malignancy, she says. Call as needed.

Additional Story, Additional History

For a year, she has had unusual tongue pain and has seen many medical and dental specialists for it. None has been able to discover the cause, and various treatments for the pain have failed. Now she has had a biopsy to look for malignancy, and she called to bring me up to date.

The Issues

- What are the causes of tongue pain in general?
- What is the cause of *her* tongue pain?

The Doctor-Patient Relationship

- H Despite the lack of a definable answer to her problem, she has not panicked. From our long relationship, she knows that I am interested, that I continue to seek an answer, that I am committed to her comfort, and that she can call me at any time and I will respond. She calls only rarely.
- H Because of the durability of our relationship, she is better able to tolerate the discomfort.

What Did I Learn?

- H In the absence of an answer, sometimes the best course is to allow more time to elapse.
- H In a trusting relationship, patients can better tolerate uncertainty.
- H An important part of being a primary care physician is providing oversight. It is important to have patients check back with information from other physicians, in order for the primary care physician to be certain that necessary tests have been completed and that the patient has had adequate explanation and an opportunity to address any unanswered questions.

Patient 11: S.T., Age 46

The Note

Abnormal liver tests: Gamma GT done 3 days ago was 67. The trend is certainly not getting worse and is better than last time.

Exam: BP 130/80. Does not look ill. Chest: clear. Heart: regular rhythm. Abdomen: soft. Liver: not palpable.

The liver test abnormality is probably of no clinical significance. No further follow-up seems warranted. Recheck in a year.

Wart: She has a wart on her finger for which she is using Compound W and has some dry skin on her fingers for which she may use skin moistener.

Additional Story, Additional History

The liver test abnormality appeared on a blood chemistry examination done at the time of her recent physical examination. She has no symptoms to suggest hepatitis or gallstones, is on no medication, and does not abuse alcohol, all potential causes of this abnormality.

The Issues

- What is the cause of the liver test abnormality? Is it of significance? Will a disease, of which this may be an early sign, later appear in a full-blown state? In the absence of an answer, what is the next step—liver biopsy, for instance, or watchful waiting? How concerned should the physician be? How concerned should the patient be?

The Doctor-Patient Relationship

- **H** I present the data, along with an interpretation and a context in which she can deal with the information. The relationship helps.

What Did I Learn?

- Abnormal test results may not necessarily indicate disease. Even if a specific disease is present, it often improves without specific treatment.
- Sometimes the physician sees a patient at the end of an illness, the major part of which caused few or no symptoms.

Patient 12: U.V., Age 58 (Telephone)

The Note

Elevated cholesterol: I spoke with her about her elevated cholesterol and will send her a diet. Recheck lipid profile in 3 months.

Nodules: She had the nodules excised and they were benign.

Additional Story, Additional History

In the past, she has had episodes of rapid heartbeat and now has the cholesterol problem. While she lives with her husband, they have been estranged for many years.

The Issues

- Not all patients with blood cholesterol elevations require drug treatment. In light of her prior heart problem, how vigorously should I treat the cholesterol elevation, if at all?

The Doctor-Patient Relationship

- H Because of her estrangement from her husband, I have a more important role in providing emotional and moral support.
- H With regard to the nodules, part of our mutual responsibility is keeping each other informed, especially of outside consultation.

What Did I Learn?

- H Problems that may seem trivial to the physician may be of major importance to the patient.

Patient 13: W.X., Age 58 (Telephone)

The Note

We reviewed the instructions of yesterday. May stop Lactinex if stools firm up.

Additional Story, Additional History

For years, the patient has had diabetes with many complications, including impaired circulation and an infected leg ulcer, for which I referred him to a surgeon. The antibiotic treatment for the leg ulcer caused the diarrhea, yet one more difficulty. He had been noncompliant with his diabetes treatment. He had a myocardial infarction years ago. He lives alone.

The Issues

- How will the diarrhea affect the control of the diabetes? Will he need an adjustment in the insulin dose?
- Are there other possible causes of the diarrhea? What are the best tests, and how urgent is it to determine that?

The Doctor-Patient Relationship

- **H** We have a long-standing relationship, and so he feels comfortable with my advice that the best test now for the cause of the diarrhea is the test of time.

- **H** Some time ago, we had recognized that his noncompliance with the diabetes treatment regimen was a compromise in his ideal care. It no longer intrudes in our transactions.

- **H** Even though he does not know the surgeon to whom I had referred him, he is comfortable with that referral because he trusts my judgment.

What Did I Learn?

- We need not do the definitive diagnostic tests for each new problem if we can make a valid educated guess, the likelihood of overlooking a disease that requires specific treatment is small, and the danger of delay in treatment, even if we have made an error, is small.

- **H** Trust can be transferable—in this case, to a surgeon.

Patient 14: Y.Z., Age 72

The Note

Polymyalgia rheumatica: Muscle and joint aching persist. He feels as bad as when he entered the hospital in December. On prednisone 8 mg a day.

Exam: BP 140/80, P 80. Does not look acutely ill. He is cushingoid.

Hemoglobin: 13.6. Sedimentation rate: 4. Electrolytes, renal function tests OK.

Increase prednisone to 10 mg daily. Prescription for 5-mg tabs, #60, 2 each a.m. Call in 6 days.

Additional Story, Additional History

The story of his muscle and joint symptoms is complex. Superimposed upon a decade of pain from osteoarthritis, degeneration of his knee, ankle, and foot joints, was a sudden worsening of the symptoms, and the additional diagnosis of polymyalgia rheumatica was made. He has hypertension. He has been depressed for years, lives alone, and does not get along well with an ill older brother, to whom he feels an obligation to provide care.

The Issues

- How do I decide on the correct dose of prednisone—by the level of pain and stiffness, by laboratory tests, or both?

- To what extent will the prednisone adversely affect the blood pressure and the depression?

The Doctor-Patient Relationship

- H As I alter the dose of prednisone from week to week, he tolerates the absence of immediate relief because he trusts my prediction of a good outcome.
- H I provide him other emotional support that helps to avoid an exacerbation of the depression.

What Did I Learn?

Even though a patient's symptoms may seem no different, sometimes a new illness with similar symptoms supervenes. We need to be aware of this phenomenon, to avoid overlooking an additional diagnosis.

Patient 18: D.E., Age 88 (Telephone–Nurse)

The Note

All in all, doing well after hernia surgery. Bladder catheter has been removed, and he is voiding adequately.

Additional Story, Additional History

The patient is intact intellectually and despite long-standing metastatic prostate cancer feels well in general. Whatever pain he has from the cancer is controlled with mild pain medicine. He lives at a nursing home, where he has found a community of other residents and staff.

The Issues

- H Should decisions about his overall care be affected by the presence of the widespread cancer?

The Doctor-Patient Relationship

- H If I had viewed him only as an elderly person with widespread cancer, I would have overlooked his intellectual competence and joy of living and dismissed any new illnesses as not to be treated.

What Did I Learn?

Despite widespread cancer, some patients can live comfortable lives for a long time.

Patient 20: F.H., Age 67 (Telephone)

The Note

He has a cough, which is evolving into symptoms of upper respiratory infection. Observe. Call if no better.

Additional Story, Additional History

In addition to his respiratory infection, he has chronic ulcerative colitis, for which he had surgical removal of his colon, and hypertension, for which he takes medicine. Whenever he feels even mildly ill, he worries that it may turn into something serious.

The Issues

Is this simply a "cold," which requires only symptomatic treatment, or does he have a bacterial infection requiring treatment with an antibiotic? How would the antibiotic affect his intestinal tract?

The Doctor-Patient Relationship

- **H** I reassure him. Our relationship validates the reassurance.

What Did I Learn?

- **H** Often, all patients need, rather than a remedy, is reassurance that their symptoms are not indicative of a serious illness.

Patient 21: G.I., Age 78

The Note

Abdominal pain, colitis: She is feeling much better. She is having three bowel movements a day and she says they are more formed than before. She will shortly stop vancomycin.

Exam: BP 130/80, P 92. Does not look acutely ill. Chest: clear. Heart: regular rhythm. Abdomen: soft, nontender. Normal bowel sounds.

Continue azulfidine. She is to call in a week with progress. If no better, may consider specific antisalmonella treatment.

Additional Story, Additional History

She is frail and elderly and lives alone. Superimposed on Crohn's disease, a chronic inflammatory disorder of the small and large intestines, and following treatment with an antibiotic for bronchitis, she developed diar-

rhea. The test for antibiotic-associated colitis from the *Clostridium difficile*
bacterium is positive.

The Issues

- Was the diarrhea caused by the recent antibiotic treatment for bronchitis,
  tainted food, a worsening of her underlying bowel inflammation, or a combination of one or more of these causes?

The Doctor-Patient Relationship

- H I drew on the "trust account" of our long relationship as I proceeded stepwise
  over several days to address the diagnosis and oversee treatment.

What Did I Learn?

- Diarrhea has many causes and may be multidetermined.
- Sometimes the treatment for one disease makes another disease worse.

Patient 22: H.J., Age 74

The Note

Hypertension: no headaches. No dizziness. On Vasotec, 2.5 mg daily.
Exam: BP 140/80. Does not look ill. Continue Vasotec, 2.5 mg daily.
Abnormal prostate: He is anticipating prostate biopsy in a week and has
a number of questions about the implications should malignancy be found
and about the approach of his urologist. We discussed all of these issues at
length.
Constipation: in the last month. Likely of no clinical consequence. He
had colonoscopy 3 months ago. Prune juice seems to help.
Return 3 months.

Additional Story, Additional History

Besides the above problems, he has had surgery for colon cancer.

The Issues

- What is the cause of the abnormal prostate? In particular, is it malignant?
- H What meaning does this have to him, particularly in light of his prior malig-
  nancy?
- H What is all this like for his wife?
- H The urologist is a new referral for him, and so he has yet to develop trust in
  his skills and advice.

The Doctor-Patient Relationship

- **H** My relationship with him and my familiarity with the urologist with whom I have worked before allow me to encourage the patient's confidence in the urologist. I assure the patient that I will be involved in his hospital care and thereafter. "We will do all we can to make things turn out well," I tell him.

What Did I Learn?

- **H** Even when the technical part of the care is in someone else's hands, the primary physician plays a substantial and crucial role in caring for the patient by overseeing his care, providing explanation, and, when necessary, endorsing the consultant's recommendations.

Patient 23: I.K., Age 82 (Telephone–Nurse)

The Note

Toe ulcer: some purulent drainage. Stop the current topical application. Soak three times a day in warm water with soap. Start clindamycin, 300 mg three times a day for 10 days. Stop promptly if she has diarrhea. I will see her tomorrow.

Additional Story, Additional History

A nursing home resident, she has many complications of diabetes, which appeared during late adulthood, including impaired circulation. She already had one leg amputation that was preceded by a toe infection, and so she has reason to fear another one. She has been depressed.

The Issues

- What is the specific bacterial cause of her infection? That determines the choice of antibiotic treatment.
- What are the potential complications of the antibiotic treatment with clindamycin, a drug that may cause colitis?
- At what point should I arrange surgical consultation?
- **H** How will this new illness affect her depression?
- **H** If a second amputation is warranted, would she accept it?
- **H** Should hospitalization be considered, or should she be cared for at the nursing home?
- **H** Though she is competent, with whom in the family should I speak?

The Doctor-Patient Relationship

H I have a long relationship with her and her family, and I dealt with them on matters related to her late husband. Our relationship facilitates dealing with all the difficult decisions regarding her care.

What Did I Learn?

- Though the diabetes appeared at a later age and the blood sugar level was never very elevated, she had many circulatory complications of the disease. Vascular complications can occur independently of the interval between the diagnosis and the present and independently of the level of blood sugar elevation.

- **H** It helps to know about the life stories of nursing home patients. Whenever I assume the care of a patient whom I had not known previously, I arrange to meet with a family member to learn more of the patient's story and establish a relationship.

Patient 24: J.L., Age 61

The Note

Headaches and hypertension: They persist. In addition, he has nausea from time to time. All of these symptoms are long-standing. On his own, he continues to take an over-the-counter preparation.

Exam: BP 120/80, P 60. Does not look acutely ill. Some limitation of rotation of neck to the left. Tenderness at level of C4–5, left paravertebral area.

Continue atenolol 25 mg daily.

He wonders about referral to "neuropathologist" because of what he feels are "spasms of the blood vessels."

Head and neck ache may be due to cervical osteoarthritis. Get cervical spine x-rays. Add diazepam, 2 mg, #60, 1 four times a day. Return 2 weeks.

He has concerns about his wife, who has an ongoing sensation of "noise in her ears." He asks for her referral to the Mayo Clinic, and I suggest that she first return to her local ear specialist.

Additional Story, Additional History

An immigrant from the former Soviet Union, he is remarkably facile with English and often helps his countrypeople by translating during physician appointments. His wife is chronically ill.

The Issues

- What is the cause of his headaches? Are they related to hypertension, vascular inflammation, tension, tumor, or some other cause?

- What is the cause of his neck aches?

- H What does he mean by "spasms of the blood vessels"?

- H Is he inappropriately demanding? If he is, what does that mean?

- H To what extent does his wife's illness affect how he feels?

The Doctor-Patient Relationship

- H The effectiveness of my care depends a great deal on my establishing a relationship by attending to all of his questions.

What Did I Learn?

- Many problems are common in a physician's practice. Headache is one. Most often the underlying cause can be discovered through careful history and physical examination. Only rarely are the more complex tests, such as a CT or MRI scan, needed to rule out a tumor or other serious cause.

- H It is important to identify, acknowledge, and discuss the patient's own view of his illness. Sometimes patients have fantasies about what is going on in their bodies.

- H In the Soviet Union, people often had difficulty gaining access to adequate medical care, and so the patient had to be extremely aggressive in obtaining what he needed. Here, American doctors can misinterpret that sort of initiative as inappropriate and "demanding." I need to understand that he has not yet established trust in the American system and in me. He is no different from any patient troubled by the uncertainty of his and his wife's illness.

- H It is important to have an appreciation of the cultural background of the patient, even if the patient is not from a different country. Each patient is an individual.

Patient 25: K.M., Age 67

The Note

Hypertension: no headaches or dizziness. Feels better on Vasotec than on Calan SR and is not "tired."
Exam: BP 160/70 sitting, 160/80 standing. P 80.
Increase Vasotec to 10 mg each a.m. Return in a month.
Diabetes: Blood sugar now is 257 at 2:50 p.m. Urged to lose weight.

Additional Story, Additional History

A long-standing patient, she is obese. She is widowed and has a single adult daughter who is intermittently depressed.

The Issues

- **H** The severity and the treatment of diabetes and hypertension are often weight dependent; the lighter, the better. How aggressive should I be in urging her to lose weight? At what point do she and I recognize that her lack of attention to weight is a substantial compromise and remove it from discussion, lest it get in the way of dealing with other issues?
- Diabetes and hypertension together are sometimes caused by Cushing's syndrome, adrenal gland overactivity. Does she need investigation for the presence of this illness?

The Doctor-Patient Relationship

- **H** Our relationship allows us to address these issues of compromise as allies and to discuss them without her feeling defensive.

What Did I Learn?

- There is a potential relationship between diabetes, hypertension, obesity, and Cushing's syndrome, a disorder of the adrenal gland. I see many patients who have both diabetes and hypertension. This co-occurrence of diseases is far more common than Cushing's syndrome, and so I need to learn simple ways to diagnose the latter.

Patient 26: L.N., Age 72 (Telephone)

The Note

Constipation: We discussed her bowel problem. Milk of magnesia taken 4 days a week seems to help. On the fifth day, she has some diarrhea. Change to milk of magnesia, 15-30 cc at bedtime as needed.

Some dizziness. Change diazepam to 2 mg four times a day as needed, instead of regularly four times a day.

Additional Story, Additional History

This nursing home resident has had constipation for many years. She has had an extensive evaluation for underlying serious causes. She and I have worked together to devise a routine of medicine and diet to improve her bowel function. In addition, she has chronic back pain, coronary heart disease and coronary bypass surgery, hypertension, and chronic depression.

When she was 60, she had a stroke. She smokes. Many years ago, when I saw that she required frequent hospitalizations for undiagnosed abdominal and back pain and was no longer able to live alone, I suggested that she consider moving to a nursing home. She agreed, though she was one of the youngest residents at the time of her admission.

The Issues

- **H** What is the reason for her call today? Is it to come up with a solution, or does she simply want me to listen?

The Doctor-Patient Relationship

- **H** But for the continuity of our relationship and the perspective that it provided, I would not have recognized years ago that she could not live alone, nor could I have convinced her of her need to live in the nursing home. Once there, I continued to care for her.

- **H** Despite the absence of definitive answers to her questions, she appreciates that I simply listen and do not judge her adversely.

What Did I Learn?

- **H** Sometimes all physicians need to do is listen. It was this patient who said (chapter 4), "When I have a physician who listens, it's magic."

Patient 27: M.O., Age 49

The Note

Edema, left leg: persists and is somewhat more prominent now, with some discomfort. He continues on anticoagulation.

Exam: BP 130/80, P 80. Does not look acutely ill. Gait is normal. Left leg: 2+ edema.

He has swelling that extends up into his thigh. No appreciable pelvic pain, but lymphatic obstruction needs to be considered.

Continue current regimen. Return 2 weeks.

Additional Story, Additional History

He emigrated from South America and is fluent in English and other languages. A knee injury at work severely disrupted his life. He was a reliable worker and an effective father; after the injury, he could not work or be as much help to his teenage sons. His marriage is failing, and he is depressed. Before he saw me, he had been referred from doctor to doctor. No one seemed to be overseeing his care or attending to the psychosocial problems.

The Issues

- What is the cause of the leg swelling and the knee pain?
- H How much of what is going on in his life is affecting how he feels and his recovery?
- H How is he handling all of this?

The Doctor-Patient Relationship

- H Until now, he has had no physician say to him, "I will oversee your care and shepherd you through this process." I offer to fill that role for him and also to look beyond the acute problems and consider the psychosocial ones. I have involved a psychologist in his care.

What Did I Learn?

- H Especially when the patient does not seem to be improving as promptly as we would anticipate, we must look beyond the obvious problems and explore psychosocial issues.

END OF THE DAY

At the end of the office day, I return to the hospital to see one of my patients for a second time. Then I go home to my family.

Patient 28: N.P., Age 45

The Note

In the evening, I receive a telephone call from the husband of a 40-year-old woman. He tells me, "She's talking and she's not making any sense." On the way to their home, I begin thinking about what might be wrong with her. (See Case 2 in chapter 10 for a discussion of this patient.)

Like most of my practice days, this one was complex and fascinating. I started at 7:30 a.m., was home by 6 p.m., and the evening's house call took an hour. During most of my practice years, I shared night and weekend call with three other internists. Because I had developed and refined a routine to what I do, a method of inquiry and interaction, and an efficient, reproducible way of looking at each problem and patient, I rarely felt rushed. I hope none of my patients did either. Practically every encounter was an opportunity for me to learn.

Medical practice is complicated, but when we truly know how to do it, most of the tasks are easy. It is easy when we can analyze the problem, identify its elements, understand how they relate to each other, come up with the best answer, work efficiently, and explain it in a way that is clear. It is tough when each decision is a struggle, as if we are dealing with it for the first time. It is easy when we learn from experience. It is easy to be a physician when we like people and get along with them; it is tough for people always getting into a scrape.

It is easy if we can organize the day, despite its inherent unpredictability; it is hard if every unscheduled demand throws us into disarray. When I worked as a busboy in a Catskill Mountains resort, my "teacher," a dental student who had worked in the resorts for many years, advised me, "Don't ever go into the kitchen empty-handed. If you're going into the kitchen to pick up an order, take some dirty dishes with you, so you can save steps and save time." Applied to daily medical practice, this means: Organize your day so that it runs efficiently. Return phone calls to patients throughout the day rather than leaving them until the end of the day. Dictate notes between patients' office visits when the information is fresh rather than at the end of the day when the memory of the transaction is more remote and the ability to concentrate wanes.

Many know this quintessential New York City story:

Tourist to native New Yorker: How do you get to Carnegie Hall?

Native New Yorker: Practice, practice, practice.

How does one get through a day of a medical career? Routines, routines, routines. Routines for approaching patients' symptoms, treating diabetes, addressing the question, "What's the cause of the patient's abdominal pain?" making a referral to a difficult-to-reach specialist. Unless our routines work—providing consistent ways of looking at illnesses, patients, and logistics—we will move through the day very slowly. The best routines include time set aside to ask, after each patient encounter, "What did I learn?"

Much of medicine *is* routine, but even the routine parts are fascinating. There are also diagnostic "highs," when we figure out an illness, the treatment for which is crucial, or one that occurs only rarely, or has been overlooked by other physicians, or one with subtle findings. There are treatment highs when, but for the physician, the patient would have died or become severely disabled. Successfully treating acute pulmonary edema or overwhelming infection are such times. Though surgeons have more of these moments, much of their work is less dramatic. Vascular surgeons operate on patients with ruptured aneurysms, but they also see patients with varicose veins. Orthopedists may deliver traffic accident victims from disaster by repairing their bones with complex emergency surgery, but they also see patients with chronic back pain.

There are "lows" also. Mistakes are a low, as I discussed in chapter 15. The death of a patient is always a loss, but not necessarily a low moment. More often it can be an especially enriching time for the physician and an opportunity to provide important support and comfort for survivors. Fatigue, from insufficient sleep or a succession of long days, is a low. The remedy is obvious—a good night's sleep, a day off. Unappreciative and angry patients are a low, but they are rare; and to the real professional, they become a challenge to discover the cause of the anger.

Then there is the human side, not so dramatic—the events in everyday practice, regardless of the physician's specialty or interests. Physicians encounter many such profound moments: the opportunity to shepherd patients and their families through a difficult illness, even one with a poor outcome, often over a period of years; the opportunity to help transform angry, isolated patients into more even-tempered people who can enter into fulfilling relationships; the opportunity to help heal broken marriages by getting husbands and wives speaking to each other meaningfully, . . .

And the opportunity to be part of so many dramas.

PART V

TEACHING THE HUMAN SIDE OF MEDICINE

Chapter 23

Teaching the Human
Side of Medicine

"If you plan for a year, sow rice. If you plan for a decade, plant trees. If
you plan for a lifetime, train and educate people."
—Chinese proverb

When students learn about the human side of medicine, the community of
patients is the ultimate beneficiary. Taking my clue from Chaim Potok
(chapter 18), I sometimes say to students:

All beginnings are hard. There are frustrations to learning. You can't understand
everything immediately, and so much bears repetition. You are learning a new way
of understanding illness and what it's like to be a patient and a physician. What is
more, as you gain knowledge and experience, you'll be on your own. Experience requires learning at every opportunity and integrating what you learn with what you
already know. That's not easy at first, and the responsibility of the teacher is to
teach you how; your responsibility is to recognize the importance of the process.

A teacher needs to be warm, welcoming, encouraging, and perceptive.
Teaching touches "the raw nerves of faith"[1]—values, in other words. As
teachers, we need to recognize the sophistication of what we do and try to
see through our students' eyes. When it is appropriate, a good physician
will say to patients, "You'll be all right soon." To students, a good teacher
will say, "Well intended and focused properly, you'll soon learn what you

need to know to be a good doctor." The partnership between student and teacher sustains the excitement.

If you want to learn a subject, find a teacher. And if you *really* want to learn a subject, *become* a teacher. The opportunity and position we have as teachers of medicine give us the responsibility to do it well. Teachers not only transmit new information, but they also model ways to approach problems and develop relationships. By their example, they can teach bad, destructive lessons or wonderful, valuable ones. We need to honor good teaching no less than good cardiac surgery. We need to recognize bad teaching also, lest silence be taken as endorsement. I encourage my students to identify and reject bad teaching.

One of my former second-year medical students told our tutorial group this story.[2]

A 45-year-old man was hospitalized because of neck pain that had been present for a few weeks, but worse in the few days prior to admission. When I examined him, I noticed weakness of the shoulder muscles and numbness in his entire arm. The rest of his examination was normal, except that his body was covered with tattoos. Two days later, when I presented the patient and his story to my instructor as a patient with a possible spinal cord lesion, all the physical findings had disappeared. The instructor felt that the patient had been malingering, was critical of me for accepting the patient's story without suspicion, and told me and my eight classmates: "Don't trust people with tattoos" and "Don't trust all your patients' stories." I felt humiliated. Initially I had felt that the patient and I had a good relationship. But after that I felt embarrassed that I had been taken for a sucker, hurt that I had been betrayed by the patient, and confused by the admonition about trusting patients. I had always believed what the patient said.

Bad teaching! Worse yet, uncritiqued and uncorrected, the teacher had given his students useless and potentially harmful information, and he had set a bad example of how to relate to a patient. But even bad teaching and bad modeling can become teachable moments. Here are some of the bad lessons and some better alternatives.

Bad lesson 1: "Don't trust people with tattoos," a prejudiced statement, no more valid than an ethnic slur, and no more useful clinically either. When our view of people is tainted by prejudice, we deny ourselves the opportunity of seeing them in *all* of their dimensions. When we as physicians define someone too narrowly, we deny ourselves creative ways of looking at them and their problems, and we may deny them a correct diagnosis and remedy. People with tattoos get sick.

These are better lessons:

- His findings cannot be explained by the realities of neurological anatomy, and so we should suspect malingering, but also the psychiatric entity called "conversion reaction." Both suggest psychosocial issues.

- That the findings at the time of his first examination cleared after two days should also raise the question of a conversion reaction or malingering.

- Conversion reaction and malingering are possibilities that should be included in the differential diagnosis of any patient with the problem statements "muscle weakness and sensory loss," but they are not the *only* diagnostic considerations.

- For all these reasons, and not because he has tattoos, consider conversion reaction and malingering.

Bad lesson 2: "Don't trust all your patients' stories." There are better lessons:

- You are better off trusting the patient until proved wrong. From a patient's perspective, there may be nothing worse than not being believed.

- People who feign illness or have conversion reactions may have concurrent organic illnesses.

- Like this problem, there are other illnesses with very dramatic moments that resolve spontaneously and have an organic cause—renal colic, seizures, and transient cerebral ischemic attacks, for example.

- Sometimes the best test is the test of time. Rather than ordering more tests, which may be costly or uncomfortable, allow some time to elapse if no harm can occur from the delay. As in this case, the passage of time helped to clarify the diagnostic issues.

- Given that this person was not telling the truth, ask, "Why not? What's going on in his life?" The answers to those questions may provide useful information.

Good teachers turn a bad experience, or a bad question, into a good one, and they often expand the question. The student's recounting of the patient's story and his own experience with less-than-ideal teaching allowed us to address other issues:

- What about the long-term management of this patient? The physician can establish an alliance with this patient without saying, "I've got the goods on you." Recognizing a moment of dishonesty gives us the opportunity to confront certain nonproductive ways in which patients deal with life and help them to discover better ways of handling things.

- What is it like for an experienced physician to face being "taken for a sucker" by a patient? By helping the student address this question, I can point out that such an event happens only rarely, but that it is part of the gamut of transactions that we face in medicine.

- As a group, we looked at what it is like to "be on the spot" as a medical student and to "need to look good." While we strive for perfection in practicing medicine, we are called upon to make so many decisions in the course of a professional day that some of them are bound to be imperfect. Such decisions are rarely of consequence, but occasionally we may cause harm. We have to be able to deal with that emotionally.

The student told of one further frustration. His teacher had said, "It is unethical to talk to anyone outside the profession about professional experiences." The consensus of the group was that we can share dilemmas with trustworthy confidants, so long as we preserve confidentiality.

Good teachers teach not simply how to *accumulate* experience, the easy part, but also how to *learn from* experience and integrate new experience into judgment, discarding methods of diagnosis and treatment that do not work. Good teachers show that every transaction in medicine is a teachable moment and how to squeeze everything possible out of those moments. Eleanor Roosevelt saw that "there is no experience from which you can't learn something."[3] *Pirke Avot*, a collection of rabbinic teachings, declares, "Who is wise? The person who learns from everybody."[4]

Good teachers appreciate that different people learn in different ways and start from different places. Years ago when I started to do darkroom work, I asked a friend, a skilled photographer, to give me some pointers on darkroom technique. He so overwhelmed me with information that it was years before I returned to the darkroom. In contrast, baseball manager Whitey Herzog said of Casey Stengel, his mentor, "Like the best teachers, he gave you the big picture in little doses."[5] Good teachers discard methods of teaching that do not work, start where the student is, and speak the student's language.

TECHNIQUES OF GOOD TEACHERS

No two patients are alike. No illness is exactly the same in two patients. No two patients have exactly the same experience with the same illness; their feelings and how they deal with the illness are different. Good physicians accommodate these differences. Good teachers accommodate the differences in the ways students learn. The teacher's ultimate goal is to teach students how to be their own teachers and how to teach *their* students, their patients, and their colleagues.

We teach from personal experience. At the beginning of their careers, medical students have scant professional experience. Nonetheless, each may have experience as a patient, as the family of a patient, in various relationships, jobs, and careers, in dealing with life's dilemmas; and experiences with teachers, good and bad. We can learn a great deal from our own experience, as chapter 5 shows.

We teach in different settings. As with teachable moments, there are also many teachable settings—at the bedside, in the clinic or office, and during formal lectures and meetings. We can create teachable moments and teachable settings in practically every clinical encounter.

We teach through stories. As an intern, I rode the ambulance to the scene of a one-car collision in Minneapolis; the car had rammed a tree. The police officer at the scene informed me that when he had arrived, the man got out of his car and "started swinging," and so he handcuffed him to the steering wheel. I was preparing to inject the man with a sedative when one of my teachers wandered by, surveyed the situation, and offered his opinion: "I wonder if he's having an insulin reaction. It's 5 p.m., about the time certain kinds of insulin reach their peak activity, and maybe he's late for a meal." Instead of an injection of a sedative, I gave him an injection of concentrated sugar, and his confusion cleared. From that experience, I learned to suspect an insulin reaction whenever confusion is present and that the confusion can be subtle.

Years later, I was speaking with a visiting insurance agent just before lunchtime. He kept asking me to repeat myself because he did not quite grasp what I was trying to say. "Do you have diabetes?" I asked. "Yes." "Are you having an insulin reaction?" He was. I saw that he immediately got food. As a medical student, I had learned that the symptoms of hypoglycemia included sweating, rapid heartbeat, and confusion. But whenever I have taught about insulin reactions, I tell these stories in order to help students become more perceptive in detecting hypoglycemia. Stories are far more effective than teaching that "X percent of patients with insulin reactions have a change in mental status."

We teach by going from the general to the specific, the specific to the general, and the narrow to the broad. As teachers we ask, "What can we generalize about this case? What is unique about this case?" By going from narrow to broad, we stimulate ourselves to learn even from the mundane. It is not a big step to learn from each case. During one week of my residency, after examining my sixth patient in succession with abdominal pain from alcohol abuse, I asked myself, "Though it's likely that this patient, like the other five, has alcoholic gastritis, a common diagnosis, why doesn't he have mesenteric artery insufficiency, a rarer cause of abdominal pain?" The exercise stimulated me to read more about the subject in medical textbooks and journals.

We teach by analogy and comparison. We teach by extracting the essence, applying what we have learned to other cases, and recognizing the similarities and the differences among them. Using the actual case, we enlarge upon the disease, the symptom, or the problem. We discover what more we need to learn. We ask, "What lessons do we learn from this case that are applicable to a patient not only with the same illness but with other ones? What effect does a difference in age have? What effect does the absence of a supporting spouse have?" We ask, "What are the unknowns? Is this case exactly like another one?"

We teach by seeing patterns and making connections. Then the "bells go off" the next time we see those associations. During residency training, I encountered two patients with severe abdominal pain, each following a similar pattern: a first period of pain, followed by a "silent period," one without pain, and then more severe pain and circulatory shock because of massive irreversible bowel injury. From the medical literature, I discovered that other patients with this unusual illness, embolus to the superior mesenteric artery, followed a similar pattern. The clue to the diagnosis was to consider it when acute abdominal pain occurred in a patient with atrial fibrillation and not be deceived by the absence of pain during the silent period. The next time I saw a patient with this combination of findings, I knew what to do before the bowel was irreversibly damaged.

We teach by keeping an open mind about different ways that diseases present themselves and relationships between problems and their treatments. We continually ask, "Is there another way to look at this?"

We teach by studying mistakes. We look at both good and bad practices. We ask, "What can go wrong in diagnosis and treatment?" Writing about how he perfected his craft as an actor, Theodore Bikel observed that "the critique that follows each piece can be very helpful. So can offering critique to others, as it hones your analytical senses."[6] By defusing the threatening aspect of critique, we turn mistakes into opportunities to learn.

We teach by studying principles of reasoning simultaneously with information about specific problems and diseases. Table 23.1 provides examples.

We teach by reinforcement and repetition. Especially during the early years of training, students need to hear a lesson more than once and in different contexts.

We teach by observing the interaction, by writing, by video- or audiotaping, and by role playing. Though each has its advantages, they all can be critiqued, reread, or recomposed. I often ask my students to "write it out, as if you were talking to him," and then we critique what they have written and how they say it as they play the doctor's role. I also tell my students that

Table 23.1
Teaching Principles of Reasoning Simultaneously with Information about
Specific Problems and Diseases

Principle	Problem or disease	Chapter, page
The importance of the patient's story	Coronary heart disease	1, 3-17
Differential diagnosis	Change in mental status	10, 85-86
	Abdominal pain	10, 82-84
The problem-oriented system	Diabetes mellitus	10, 88-92
Seeing patterns, making connections	Superior mesenteric artery embolus	23, 222

I will closely critique the quality of their written work because I believe that how they write reflects the clarity of their thinking.

We teach by modeling. I know a master trumpeter who invites his students to his performances and encourages them to watch others perform. One of my colleague's students told me, "I was in a tough situation, and I asked myself, 'What would Bill [his teacher] say in this situation?' "

And so a teaching encounter may integrate many of these principles.

- One student presents a case, the summary of the patient's story (the history) and the physical examination.
- While the student presents the story, another constructs a problem list for all to see.
- The students and the teacher critique and sharpen the precision of the problem list by asking: "Is the problem list complete? Have all the problems been properly named?"
- The students and the teacher validate and enhance the history by returning to the patient for additional details to answer the questions defined by the above steps. The teacher models the process by interviewing the patient in the students' presence.
- The students and the teacher continue the discussion by talking further about the patient, the diseases, the problems yet undefined, issues of the doctor-patient relationship, and tactics for diagnosis and treatment.

- And then they ask, "What did we learn?"

In each of these steps, the teacher can see where students are in their comprehension and reasoning and move them along at their own pace. "A student has the right to be challenged," one student wrote.

The best teachers like what they are doing. And they like their students.

The best teachers understand their subject. They know the best techniques for teaching it and can describe them. They teach with clarity of presentation, purpose, and intent. They ask clear questions and follow with "Do you understand?" From medical school and postgraduate residency training, I still remember that whether the feverish child *looks* ill is often more important than how high the temperature is. I also remember not only who taught me these lessons, but when and where I learned: the "silhouette sign" in chest x-rays, how to interpret a blood sodium level, the differential diagnosis of pulmonary edema, and the best way to examine a thyroid gland.

The best teachers use common sense, common nonphysician sense. Technical knowledge adds to thoughtful decisions, but rules can sometimes get in the way of original thinking if we do not understand where they apply. I teach, "Never do anything that violates your common sense."

The best teachers use their "personality." They are part of their message. "Preaching," a minister friend and patient recognized, is "the bringing forth of truth through personality." One need not be garrulous, but simply genuine. Good salespeople sell their product by selling themselves.

If all these qualities of a good teacher seem familiar, it is because they are qualities of a good physician. While I do not regard my students as patients, I recognize that, as a teacher, I use many of my physician skills. There is one more analogy.

The teacher-student relationship is like the doctor-patient relationship. One way to explore the doctor-patient relationship is to use the teacher-student relationship as a model. I ask students, "What are you, as a student, entitled to ask of your teachers? What are you, as a patient, entitled to ask of your physician?" I urge them to examine ways in which the two relationships are similar. I also ask them to compare our relationship at our first session with our later one, well into the semester, and to see how time enhances both relationships. The analogy works.

The best teachers develop a relationship with their students. With the relationship comes trust, respect, candor, and consistency. You cannot learn from someone you do not trust, and teachers need to trust their students. Continuity provides the teacher with awareness of students' own stories and fund of knowledge; teachers can encourage students who are frustrated or moving slowly because they know why. The best teachers are accessible and approachable.

PHYSICIANS LEARN FROM THEIR PATIENTS

Our patients are our faculty. Not from a teacher or a text, but from patients, I learned that pneumonia and congestive heart failure can cause confusion and that patients with coronary artery insufficiency may not have chest pain but only shortness of breath. I have also learned big-picture lessons: that people can cope with illness in many ways and that almost any drug can cause almost any side effect. Better than any text, patients teach us various ways that illnesses manifest themselves. From patients I learned what it is like to *be* a patient. From a friend with cancer, I learned that being examined in a gown "dehumanizes" her, and so she now negotiates with her physician to examine her in street clothes.

From patients I also learned what *not* to say. We cannot possibly choose every word, and even ordinary transactions can be complicated. But we can learn from every transaction. To a young patient with pancreatitis, alcoholism, depression, and seizures, I said, as encouragement, "Our goal is to get you back to where you were [in life, before this acute illness]." But he responded, "I need acceptance for where I *am*." He explained that because of his diseases, multiple medications, and multiple physicians' appointments, he could never get back to where he was, and my statement simply gave him another unattainable goal. A better goal, he suggested, was to get to "as good as it can be."

To comfort someone after the death of her spouse, I said, "I know how you feel." "You can't possibly know how I feel," she responded with a hint of outrage. I learned quickly. Now in similar situations I say, "I can only begin to appreciate how you must feel."

From patients' stories, we learn that illnesses, acute or chronic, poke along sometimes, and when the answers became more clear, we wonder, "Why didn't we figure this out sooner?" But that is the way life is in general: Decisions poke along, and only toward the end do we see the solution that was staring us in the face and gain new insights.

From patients, we learn that congestive heart failure sometimes persists because of ongoing dietary salt indiscretions, controlling the blood sugar level in diabetes sometimes is difficult because the patient cannot see the markings on the insulin syringe, and controlling high blood pressure sometimes fails because the patient cannot afford the medicine and is too embarrassed to say so.

We learn from families, who are often far more expert on the subtleties of an illness than their physicians. An 80-year-old woman's children detected a subtle change in her mental status that I had overlooked. That led to a diagnosis of subdural hematoma, a blood clot pressing on the brain, curable with surgery.

Sometimes we see successes and extraordinary recoveries that we cannot explain. From patients, we learn why. An initially grim prognosis was inaccurate because the diagnosis was in error, the problem was not so precisely defined, or because some people simply defy the odds. The person whom the physician feared discharging from the hospital managed quite well because the patient was more resourceful than the physician thought.

A giant leap in the physician's maturity occurs when we make the transition from learning *about* our patients to learning *from* them. An undergraduate discovered early that "the patient's illness provides a focal point for a new learning experience in which the physician and patient use their experiences to learn from each other."

Of the evolution of the teacher-student relationship and its parallel with the doctor-patient relationship, an undergraduate wrote:

Before taking this seminar course, I had no idea who you were or anything about you. . . . Even though I am still wary speaking in class, I have become more comfortable because you value everyone's opinion and story. You ask probing questions and seem interested in what everyone has to add to class discussion. . . . I feel the job of a teacher is to guide students along their journey of learning. . . . Teachers take on many forms throughout an individual's life. Some may be mentors, educators, friends, advocates, counselors, or encouragers. . . . [The student-teacher relationship] is one which concentrates on personal growth. . . . One must realize the limitations a physician and teacher are working under as well as student and patient. Both professionals must be very observant and recognize subtle clues that lead the teacher to a "teaching" diagnosis and the physician to a "health" diagnosis.

All physicians are teachers. Not all physicians teach students, but all teach patients. A third-century Chinese proverb declares, "If you plan for a year, sow rice. If you plan for a decade, plant trees. If you plan for a lifetime, train and educate people."[7] We are teaching how to learn and how to become our own teacher. Part of the Hippocratic Oath is our obligation to teach. Each of us—physicians, teachers, students, and patients—has much to teach; we need only examine our experiences. The goal of a good teacher is to help make the lessons explicit and pass them on. Being a teacher has all the qualities and responsibilities of being a physician: the intensity, the continuity, the relationship—and the satisfaction.

PART VI

SUMMING UP

Chapter 24

Fashioning the Best System of Medical Care Possible: What Would Be Ideal for the Patient; What Would Be Ideal for the Physician

"Good medicine does not just happen; it is thoughtfully planned and practiced."

Throughout this book, the voices of patients have expressed what they need from their physicians and from the system of medical care. Young and without professional experience, my students at Macalester College developed their own ideas about what is ideal for the patient *and* for the doctor, for unless physicians are happy in their work, both they and their patients suffer.

The students' final assignment in the course each year is "to write a term paper on 'Fashioning the best system of medical care possible: what would be ideal for the patient; what would be ideal for the physician.'" I tell them that I am not asking them to detail a "national health care system." Rather they should "describe what you, as a patient, would seek from your physician and from a system of health care, and what you, as a physician, would want in a career to which you have dedicated yourself." I ask them to draw on many sources—the content of their reading and classroom discussions for the seminar, but also their own experience, feelings, and wisdom. I tell them that in this essay, I want to get some sense of their values.

In the assignment for this paper, I remind them that "medicine must be sufficiently attractive to bring talented, bright, compassionate, thoughtful men and women to a career that is, on the one hand, stimulating, satisfying, and intellectually challenging and, on the other, requires many years of training, a continuing commitment to learning, and a substantial invest-ment of time and money in education."

I am proud of their insights and reflections. They complement those of patients and experienced physicians. They validate my view that the es-sence of the human side of medicine is present in them all. Here are some eloquent excerpts.

WHAT WOULD BE IDEAL FOR THE PATIENT

This student essay provides a nice context.

Each of us faces moments when our reality becomes unrecognizable, our security weakens, and our choices no longer follow a familiar path. For many, it is illness that shatters this world of comfort, security, and certainty. When we become ill, we lose control over the functions and care of our physical being. Our weakness forces us to ask others for assistance, and . . . we must depend on the knowledge and skills of others to restore our health. This dependence creates a unique relationship be-tween the ill and the healer. We turn to healers when we no longer recognize the language of our body—we ask that they listen, understand, and respond to our body's demands. In all communities, throughout all cultures, the healer, therefore, is a valuable and well respected member. The relationship between healers and their patients relies on the skill, knowledge, and dedication of the healer and yet is centered on the needs and story of the patient. It is this balance that remains fun-damental in the ideal relationship between the ill and their healers. . . .

Physicians are not asked to plunge into an endless series of medical interven-tions and therapies; we don't ask them to continue treatment no matter what the consequence or never to fail. Instead, we ask physicians to listen to our choice of paths, our personal history, and our glimpse of the future. We ask that they never forget who we are and that they treat us as individuals. In asking for this under-standing, we ask for far more of physicians than simply their technical talents. We ask that they incorporate their personal judgments, skills, and opinions, with our expectations—that together we create the most effective plan of treatment. In this manner, we maintain the balance of our relationship. The focus remains on the pa-tient and all decisions are products of shared expectations and values.

Patients appreciate simple humanity. Another student saw her long-time personal physician as a model.

She was recommended to me by a friend. Once she entered, the room suddenly lit up. She had a warm smile, a caring look, and enthusiasm to see me. She gracefully approached me and shook my hand while introducing herself. I forgot for a moment that I was ill and instead was in amazement. She set an atmosphere that was comfortable. She treated me with so much care and most of all respect. She listened to my story, without writing any words on paper, and asked questions only when there was a pause. She examined me with care and had a correct diagnosis. I felt I could tell her anything, that I could trust her. It had only been a matter of minutes, and I wanted to tell her my life. After that appointment I was happier than I had been for a long time and made it a priority that I have her as my personal doctor. That is a doctor that every patient is entitled to.

Patients want the right to choose. Another wrote:

My first demand is that I should have the right to choose my physician. The qualities that I would search for in my ideal doctor would be medical astuteness, personable style, and concern about all aspects of my personal health, including my physical condition, my emotional state, and my psychological well-being. A physician who could respond to me personally would be perfect.... [In a complex medical situation] I would like my physician to be my counselor, as well as the orchestrator, organizer, and conductor of all the specialists to whom I may be referred. [Such a physician] would be essential to my sense of security that everything is being coordinated in a manner that seems reasonable to someone who knows both the medical requirements of the situation, and the needs that I pose as an individual.

Patients want a relationship and understanding. As one student suggested:

The best health care system is one that should model after the family.... The relationship between the parent and the child is a delicate one. Even though the parent and the child are from the same family, they experience life differently because of age, sex, or other factors. In order for understanding to take root and the family to work together as a unit, each person must listen and be listened to. This is the same interaction that must occur in a doctor's office, because doctors and patients come from different worlds. They have their own backgrounds. They live their own lives.

Physician and patient need to like each other. One of my students wrote of her doctor, "I liked him from the start, and I felt that he liked me as well, which mattered a lot.... It never occurred to me that [he] even had patients other than me.... I never felt that I had to handle anything alone, including the uncertain future of my condition."

Patients want a partnership with their physician. One student described some aspects of that partnership.

Collaboration between doctors and patients is important to the patient and to the relationship. It empowers patients and makes them active members in determining their future; and it attests to the doctor's trust of the patient's judgment. Collaboration indicates to patients . . . that doctors think of them as individuals . . . that physicians realize that although the patient may have the same sickness as someone else, he is also unlike anyone else in that he requires his own treatment. . . .

The doctor-patient relationship is similar to a business deal sealed with a handshake. There is no written agreement that the doctor will always be available to answer questions, no clause stating that the doctor must present every treatment available to the patient, no law guaranteeing that the doctor will even be willing to collaborate on a treatment with a patient. Yet, in a successful doctor-patient relationship, all these things are present because of an established mutual trust and respect between the physician and the patient.

Another student recognized other unique qualities of the partnership.

Doctors work as the "expert" on the technical, medical part of the problem, and patients work as the "expert" on the lifestyle and context parts of the problem. Of course, the boundary between the two roles is not (and should not be) completely clear. The doctor may have recommendations for lifestyle changes, and the patient may have opinions or insights regarding possible treatments. Nevertheless, these two "experts" come together and inform each other of the various aspects within their areas of expertise.

Though one student said it differently, she appreciated the unique partnership, in which the patient is not passive.

Although it is doctors who have been educated in the anatomy and physiology of the human body and in the diagnosis of ailments, it is patients who live in the body and relate this body to the world. Therefore, it should be the role of patients to share what they know as the long-time owner and inhabitant of the body and the role of physicians to apply this information to their academic knowledge in exploring and making a diagnosis. Thus, it is vital that patient and physician together discuss what they know so a complete diagnosis and understanding of the illness as a whole can be obtained. In the process of exchanging information, a relationship between patient and physician develops, allowing both life worlds to overlap in a wealth of information and insight used to make a more complete diagnosis. . . . Patients should ultimately be the co-creator of their own medical treatment, using physicians' medical expertise to make safe, satisfying health care decisions unique to their individual needs.

Sometimes patients need authorization to tell their story and to be honest about their feelings. If patients are reticent, it is the physician's responsibility to assist them through thoughtful inquiry. Encouraging patients to be forthcoming regarding information and feelings adds to the quality of the story. One student recognized that

many people don't tell the truth, or don't relate all their symptoms because they aren't comfortable telling such personal stories. They feel as if they must be the only one [who has such a story]—or that it is "bad" for them to be feeling the way that they are. Different people have varying levels of comfort within a doctor's office, and this can often be noticed in the telling of their stories. I think being naive, unaware, or ignorant of important symptoms can also be a problem for patients. Many people just don't know—or suspect, but think their suspicions are ungrounded—and don't relate crucial symptoms or happenings to their physicians.

Patients want their physicians to listen. They want to tell their story and have sufficient time to do it. Another student tried to plumb the feelings of a mythical patient, when he wrote:

It feels very frightening to think that a doctor can confuse a patient's diagnosis because he or she doesn't have time to listen. That "well-known" doctor became "ill-known" for me. He didn't possess the patience to listen to my story. Perhaps telling stories was the only time where I felt I was in control, but that doctor took this satisfaction away from me. . . . How could he go on and say this particular kind of treatment is appropriate in my case when he didn't know my whole story?

Patients want empathy. Students reinforced the idea that patients want their doctors to appreciate what it is *like* for them and to understand that illnesses and people are complex. One wrote, "I want the medical system and my physicians to see . . . the humanism of [my illness and that even] a rational person can do that which is not in his or her best interests. . . . I don't want my physician to conclude that if I am not doing well, it's because I'm bad, i.e., 'noncompliant.' I'm just having a hard time."
Another observed that

physicians should . . . try to understand what it is like to go through the illness from the patient's perspective, of being ill in a world full of prejudices and generalizations based solely on appearances. Social stigmas accompany any illness; and with illness that may affect patients' physical appearance or ability, the stigmas can be especially harmful. Cancer patients who go through chemotherapy and lose their hair know that this is a side effect of the chemicals used, but may not be mentally prepared for having everyone look and know that they have cancer. Illness is a very private matter. . . . Physicians who are honest about what is at stake relay the message that they understand some of the silent concerns about going through the illness. By being honest with a patient and not covering up some of the emotionally detrimental aspects of an illness, a doctor can begin establishing trust with his patient.

One student elaborated on physicians' unique position to validate patients' experiences and feelings. "Doctors should be able to acknowledge that patients' discomfort and/or illness are crises in their lives, not just another addition to the doctor's rounds. . . . I think that it is unrealistic and undesirable for physicians to become every patient's personal counselor, but by merely acknowledging the emotions accompanying illness, doctors communicate to patients that they empathize and see them as human beings."

One wrote simply, "The quality of compassion in a physician should not be a bonus, it should be a prerequisite."

In their physicians, patients need original thinkers. That student also observed that "the physician should be innovative; he or she should know how to examine problems from all different angles and consider new solutions."

Patients need physicians who recognize that technology alone is not always the answer. One student saw that "the existence of powerful medical technology doesn't mean one must do away with more 'old-fashioned techniques,' most notably careful history taking and clinical judgment, [which] can provide information that a CT scan or blood test cannot. . . . An understanding of the real problem, and the most effective treatment for it, is [often] not even touched on by a test, but is arrived at, rather, by human insight." He was concerned about what technology could come to symbolize for some patients.

Certainly CT scans, laparoscopy, blood tests, and the like can symbolize safety and certainty to patients. But in talking to people and recalling some of their feelings about their doctors, I also get the sense sometimes that the use of these types of tests at the same time symbolizes something cold . . . and inhuman about the practice of medicine to some patients. Tests are designed to measure biological variables relevant to disease. But more often than not, these same measurements are what seem to be of the least essence to the patient. If tests are not balanced by a thoughtful consultation and history-taking by the doctor, the patient may get the feeling that the doctor's main interest in these seemingly mysterious measurements means the patient and his experience have been fundamentally misunderstood.

The ability to deal with emotional issues should be part of the armamentarium of each physician. One student observed that "individualizing treatment and humanizing medicine . . . requires that physicians address the emotional difficulties faced by persons who are ill. For this to occur, the doctor must listen well and be especially perceptive of the unspoken words." Another recognized that "the commitment to handling the deeply felt emotions of patients and caregivers cannot be dismissed as someone else's responsibility. Dealing with the patient's emotions is not a peripheral task of the physician. Rather, along with controlling the disease process, it should be one of the physician's main objectives."

Patients want adequate explanation. Still another student cited the need for enough information in understandable language.

Illnesses are difficult situations that are only complicated by stress, confusion and complex medical terminology. As a result, I believe that I would greatly appreciate an attentive physician who was willing to explain the illness and its possible consequences in a clear, open, and honest manner. . . . In a time of fear and uncertainty, clear and complete information is absolutely necessary. . . . My ideal doctor would serve as a "guide" or "translator" throughout the illness, functioning as someone who could inform me about what to expect and assist me in making complex medical decisions.

In their physicians, patients need teachers. One student realized the many dimensions to that role. "As teachers, doctors can reach out to the families and serve as supporters of the family's struggle by providing context and information. To patients, they can act as knowledgeable guides on the path of illness, showing them where the pitfalls are and how best to avoid or survive them."

There are many dimensions to healing. Patients need them all. Another student's questions and insights about healing and the dimensions of medicine beyond the technical were shaped in part by her father, a minister.

I grew up thinking about medicine and healing from a spiritual as well as a physical perspective. . . . Healing . . . as in the case of a chronic or terminal illness means coming to terms with the pain and what is to come. . . . Healing asks for the support of other people, and this support system can be an area of brokenness in people's lives. Healing involves learning how to better communicate with loved ones, so that each person's needs are fulfilled and dreams understood. . . .

To be artfully, humanly competent . . . is what distinguishes a good physician from a great one. [Competence is] built upon the foundation of patient-centered care and policies, effective communication, awareness of the familial, societal, and medical context in which illness and health care take place, and a sense of the profound. *Good medicine does not just happen; it is thoughtfully planned and practiced. . . .* [Italics mine]

Illness, especially serious and terminal illness, often causes people to rethink the course of their lives and reexamine goals and what is ultimately important. The physician is in a privileged position to share these moments with patients.

WHAT WOULD BE IDEAL FOR THE PHYSICIAN

One student's observations provide the context. In essence, they are about values. His father, a cardiac surgeon, is his model and teacher.

My father told me once that he was trained as "a technician," but he emerged "a healer."... I realized... that it was not his job that he placed above everything else, but the people whom he served—his patients. I understood then the true humanism of medicine. . . . The practice of medicine today consolidates the two disciplines of science and art—the science of technology and the art of healing. . . . This doctor-patient partnership is the foundation of the art of healing. . . .

The privilege afforded physicians is to be a part of the lives of other people. . . . What can be learned from treating patients contributes to the physician's professional and personal growth. . . . If a physician can see the patient as a valuable resource—if the physician will search for the truth of the illness in the patient's story—only then will the patient best be served. Through all of this comes the reward of practicing medicine.

Physicians need time. Another student wrote that "as a physician, I would desire a medical system that would allow me to be the kind of doctor that I want to be. . . . I would want to have the time necessary to get to know each patient as an individual . . . the freedom to organize my own time and choose how many patients I am going to see."

Physicians need a learning, intellectually challenging, and collaborative environment. A student described her goal as

a learning environment where I can establish mutually beneficial relationships with patients and co-workers. Learning is a continual process, and being a physician provides a unique opportunity to learn from people's unique stories and experiences. . . . Working with patients, peers, and other co-workers in a team would give me access to a problem-solving think tank. . . . I want to look back at my life and career and see where I have helped out humankind and what I have learned from my patients and my peers.

One of her classmates had similar views:

The primary care physicians are the first doctors to deal with all the problems of their patients and must perform a multitude of tasks. Collaboration is key. . . . As a physician, I would want this type of intellectual challenge, always dealing with something new and having to figure it out. Having a consortium of peers to consult would be critical as well. Not only my [physician-]partners, but schoolteachers, religious figures, nurses, families, friends; from all I would seek to learn. . . .

A diverse pool of patients would help me to recognize some of my [own] prejudices, so that I am able to work around them. . . . [From them] I would learn the variety of ways in which people heal or motivate themselves. Religion, optimism, meditation, inspirational readings, music—there are so many things in this world that people draw on to "get them through" and to stay centered. . . . Through a diverse group of patients, I would hope to learn techniques which I might apply to another patient's situation.

Physicians need the opportunity to reflect. One student would like a setting in which "we [colleagues] might discuss moral implications of certain methods of treatment, suggestions for solutions to case problems, or ideas for further resources. . . . I would like to have programs in which I would have the time to bring together people who have similar health concerns, so that they could share their experiences, and I could have a chance to teach what I can about taking care of ourselves."

Physicians need to feel comfortable in recognizing that no one is perfect; everyone makes mistakes. Another student's ideal medical system "would allow doctors to be human. This means that doctors themselves need to come to terms with their inherent fallibility as human beings. They need to be free to discuss with colleagues mistakes that they have made. . . . Both doctors and patients need to remember that being human involves grieving over mistakes and losses, and physicians should not be expected to be immune from feeling that pain." One young man hopes for "a more open environment for the physician by holding regular conversation hours in clinics and hospitals, where the physicians would sit together to discuss their stories of when they were humbled by medicine."

Benefits for the physician go beyond financial ones. Another student wrote: "In the medical field there are intellectual and social benefits that can be as attractive as economic compensation. . . . [Among these benefits are] varied opportunities to get involved in continuing education programs, . . . a supportive and fertile environment within a research community, . . . [and] accessibility to mentors and peers. The fact that problems and challenges are not always solved in the same manner opens opportunities for diverse thinking and . . . creativity."

A student described the uniqueness of the medical profession:

As one physician told me, after a while the illnesses one sees become familiar and, perhaps, no longer as interesting in themselves as they once were. But the way in which the patient experiences and describes his or her illness, on the other hand, is always unique and thus always potentially edifying. This fact is what can keep the practice of medicine interesting and fulfilling for the physician and, as a consequence, make the physician more effective and durable.

The overlap in patients' needs and those of physicians is no coincidence, and that in itself is a lesson. For both patients and physicians, the themes are recurring: simple humanity, relationship and partnership, the ability to listen and learn from each other, and the time to do it. Our ongoing task as physicians and teachers is to validate and reinforce these themes. When values such as these are present at the beginning, they are worth preserving. Patients and students should accept nothing less.

Chapter 25

Epilogue and My Personal Journey

"You do not have to be a genius to be a really good doctor. It takes a good head—and a good heart."

When I stopped practicing in 1997 after a serious illness, from which I have since recovered, I sent each of my patients a letter, which said in part:

I know it is not easy to change physicians. With many of you, the relationship that we have shared goes back many, many years. My relationship with others has been shorter. And so each of you may see this need to change physicians as more or less of a loss.

I, too, feel a loss. My career in medicine has been one of great satisfaction and joy. Many have asked me, "What is the best part of medicine for you?" and the answer is an easy one: the *relationships* with my patients. You have shared with me your stories, not only about your illnesses, but also about your lives in general, the challenges, successes, and frustrations you have faced, and how you have dealt with them. I have been touched by that trust and have learned a great deal from each of you. The wisdom that you have shared with me, I believe, has made me a better physician and teacher.

From my own recent illness, I have learned once again what I already knew about the important elements in medical care: the need for continuity, for compassion and comforting, for adequate explanation in language that is understandable, and the need for accessibility. All of this takes time, and none of this should be compromised.

There were many levels to this letter. It was a warm message to my patients and a validation of our alliance. In a few words, it was my professional credo, what I thought was important in medicine. It was authorization and encouragement to my patients to seek what I consider the best in a physician. And it was a challenge to my partners, who saw the letter, to continue to meet those standards.

Notice that I began this chapter with "When I stopped practicing" and not "When I retired." I remain an involved physician. I continue to teach, and I continue to reflect on what I have done during my career. But being a physician does not define me completely. I am a husband, a father, a son, a brother, a teacher, and a writer. Through the years, I have changed both location and direction in my career. I belong to various communities beyond the community of physicians—a community of friends, the Jewish community, the larger St. Paul community, and the Macalester College and University of Minnesota Medical School communities, among others. Being a physician gives me the opportunity to draw from, and share, many interests. Friends and family still come to me, the physician, not for care but rather for advice and direction. I can move things along, get their doctor's attention, and get them timely appointments. So should it be for all patients, even those without a connection with someone who knows how to work the system.

As a reflective person, I had always wanted to write about these things, and to ask, "Can they be taught, or does one need personal dramatic experiences to learn them?" I started to write this book several years ago, while I was still practicing. Now I really have the time. Obviously, there is a lot of me in this book. I relate my own experiences, not because they are unique, but rather because they illustrate a number of elements of a medical career. Change is a reality. Dealing with change is a necessity. Values dictate action. A career in medicine offers many opportunities. One is not simply a physician but also part of a family and a community. We do not have to handle things alone.

Much has happened to me in the course of thinking about this book over a period of years. I have developed new insights into what doctors do and how they go about doing it. I have found new questions to ask, such as "What is a professional?" One of the unexpected outcomes has been an enhancement of my perceptions about the nature of medicine and how we learn. I became even more attentive, while I practiced, to the stories and lessons from my practice, and so each day became even more exhilarating. Through the years, I kept records not only of clinical information and data but also of how people told their stories and talked about their feelings. I also recorded how I teach my students, what they say, what works, and what does not work. Writing this book has enabled me to restructure the order of what I teach and to rethink the process of teaching. I found that the process of thinking about and writing this book validated that medicine is a complex and worthy profession. It is, in a word, fascinating.

My own story is no more or less important than the story of many other physicians. Each of our stories draws on experience, models, values, and what we have learned from our patients and from life itself. I have been a patient. The story of the patient who had coronary bypass surgery (chapter 1) was my own. Members of my family have been patients. Each of my parents' serious chronic illness helped me understand, early on, the impact of illness, not only on the one who is ill but also on the person's family. At age 47, my mother discovered a lump, which turned out to be breast cancer. She died eleven years later. At the time of her diagnosis, my father was 50, my sister was 15, and I was 20. Not long after that, my father had a recurrence of a severe depression that persisted, more or less, until his death, close to his ninetieth birthday. As a family, we have experienced other illnesses, great and small, and felt the impact of those illnesses on our day-to-day existence and on our relationships.

These stories are all part of my experience, as was the intervention of our family's surgeon, Irving Cramer. As a kid, I knew nothing of his competence and would not have known how to judge it; I simply assumed that he always knew what he was doing. He remained my mentor for at least half of my career as a physician, until he died. He is still my primary model. He cared for all my family even when the issues were not surgical.

When I speak to patients, I speak with all these voices. With a depressed patient and his family, I think of my father, and I have an extra measure of understanding and compassion. With a woman with breast cancer and her family, I think of what it was like for my mother—and for my father, sister, and me. When I talk with a patient with mononucleosis, I think of my wife's experience and her relief that she had *only* mononucleosis and not the malignancy she feared. When I am dealing with a difficult situation, I ask myself, "How would Irv have handled it?" And I try never to forget to say, "Oy!"

My experience as an undergraduate at Hamilton College in upstate New York, outlined in chapter 18, deepened my appreciation of the joy of learning and the human elements. At the University of Rochester School of Medicine and Dentistry, how we learned was as important as what we learned. A gifted group of physicians trained doubly as internists and psychiatrists taught us the importance of psychological and social issues in determining the process and outcome of illness. Taught throughout the four years and on every clinical service, the biopsychosocial model was the way we looked at all patients, whether they were on a psychiatry or a surgery ward, in the clinic, or in the emergency room. When my class returns for reunions, we—internists, surgeons, and psychiatrists alike—tell each other stories of how that model has influenced our careers. To be a student at Rochester was the privilege to learn in a nurturing, supportive atmosphere.

I worked as a summer volunteer medical student at the Grenfell Mission Hospital in northern Newfoundland, where nurse-midwives provided the primary care for the people in the villages. Early in my career, they taught me the value of the nurse-physician partnership. Physicians there were jacks-of-all-trades and had multiple skills. During internship and medical residencies at Minneapolis General Hospital (now Hennepin County Medical Center) and Cleveland Metropolitan General Hospital, both public hospitals, and the Cleveland Veterans Administration Hospital, I had wise academic and community physicians as teachers and models. My residency was interrupted by a two-year stint in the U.S. Air Force, where I practiced radiology as well as internal medicine; there I began to get a taste of what it would be like to have my own practice.

I started private practice in Gloucester on Massachusetts' North Shore, 25,000 people and 25 doctors, a mix of family physicians, surgeons, pediatricians, obstetrician-gynecologists, and internists. Other specialists and subspecialists from nearby communities and Boston came to consult. My one concern in going to Gloucester was that if people became *really* sick, they would want their care in Boston, "the mecca," an hour away. As it turned out, practically no one wanted to go to Boston; patients preferred to remain in their hometown, near family and friends, cared for by their own physicians and nurses in their own community hospital. Their trust was well founded. The community of physicians was broadly skilled and devoted to patients. Only rarely did a patient have to be referred elsewhere. During my two years in Gloucester, I learned what I could do, what exceeded my skills, and what breached my threshold of concern. I learned to work efficiently and to rely on my colleagues. And whenever I found that my need for information or advice could not be satisfied with what was available locally, I would call one of my former teacher-experts from residency.

Though I had been fulfilled as a physician practicing in Gloucester, we had other needs as a family—to be close to at least one of our families of origin, to meet our religious needs more completely, and to have the cultural benefits of a larger city. And so we moved from the small town, where I was one of few physicians, to St. Paul, where I was one of many. During those years, my practice situation changed more than once. After seven years, I left a partnership and took my established practice to a new location in the same building. Though I had a solo practice, I was never alone. I always had

trusted colleagues with whom I shared night, weekend, holiday, and vacation coverage. We discussed difficult cases and decisions, and I always had
the larger medical community as a resource.

After four years, I formed a new partnership with a physician fifteen
years younger, just out of training. We quickly found that we shared ways of
viewing medical problems and dealing with patients. Most of all we shared
values. Then we merged our practice with two other offices. The sociology
of the merged office was far different from what I had envisioned, and ultimately we broke up that office and my former partner and I joined a larger
group, though we maintained our separate office. Despite the different atmosphere in the merged office and then the larger group, I tried to avoid
compromising on time and values.

Other things changed. When I started practice in St. Paul, there were
few subspecialists in internal medicine, and so I dealt with a broader range
of problems. With the arrival of more physicians who separately
subspecialized in the care of diseases of specific organ systems, we general
internists tended to see the less complicated cases as referral patterns and
patient choices changed. Yet I remained professionally satisfied, stimulated, and busy. The reality has always been that patients need physicians
who provide the broad view and continuity of primary care and who coordinate complicated care.

There were other reasons for my satisfaction. Through the years, I often
began something new. Because of my interest in the "problem-oriented system" of medical reasoning and recording, I oversaw a program of
nurse-physician collaboration at my community hospital, and I consulted
with a computer company early in the days of computer applications to
medicine. I traveled to a small town in Wisconsin once a month to provide
internal medicine consultation. I joined the editorial board of a nursing
magazine where I provide a physician's perspective on issues related to
nursing.

And I have always taught. Teaching has been an opportunity to refine
my thinking and reasoning and to "recycle" what I know. Teaching has kept
me on my toes and stimulated. I have taught medical students and residents, nurses, clergy and seminary students, undergraduates, and adults and
children in the community.

Among the perks of being a physician are these additional things I
learned:

- There is more to being a physician than technical expertise. Ask any patient.
  Ask any doctor.

- Hearing other people's stories allows me to count my own blessings and put things in perspective. When you have your health and your family, there is hardly anything else you need.
- Medicine is a metaphor for life. What we—patients and physicians—learn in dealing with illness has application outside the medical setting.
- When we neglect the human side of medicine, everyone—patients and physicians—loses.
- It is easier to learn about the human side early on—as an undergraduate and as a medical student. It is harder to learn these principles of care as a resident and harder yet once one is in practice.
- Patients do not change. What we know about illnesses does—their cause, their treatment, their prognosis. The system changes. Physicians change. Their reasons for choosing medicine as a life's work may change. Their expectations may change. Their attitudes may change. But patients do not change.
- There are lots of really good doctors around. They are not "the world's foremost authorities," but they are very, very good, technically excellent and skilled in the tasks of addressing the human side of medicine, the timeless dimensions of medical care. No patient should settle for anything less. This is not simply a yearning for "the good old days" and what can no longer be. Our task is to extract the best from each era, before and during the arrival of technology and other advances, and integrate them with what is worthwhile in the new. By doing that, physicians keep themselves balanced, renewed, and stimulated.
- There are more kindred souls out there than you can imagine. Teaching my course at Macalester has allowed me to connect with many physicians in the community who share the same feelings and values and are eager to talk about them with students and with each other. We just never found each other! And such physicians are the best recruiters for medicine.
- If we are to be satisfied in a medical career, we need to talk more about the human side of medicine. We enrich each others' lives when we do that.
- Physicians are important guardians of the values of health care. Our credential is still powerful. And our actions, as individual practitioners, are important, both for patients and for ourselves.

Among the myths about medicine are these:

- The patient has to choose a physician who has excellence in either the technical or the human side of medicine—The patient is entitled to both.
- You can forgo the relationship—You cannot. The relationship is the vehicle for most transactions between the patient and the physician.
- The relationship is important only to the patient—wrong again. It is just as important to the physician. Without it, we cannot be happy in our work, and it is important for doctors to be satisfied professionally.

- You can compromise on time—You cannot. Adequate time is crucial to all aspects of medicine, technical and nontechnical.
- You cannot have a personal life as a doctor—You can. And your personal and professional life can complement each other.

And finally, you do not have to be a genius to be a really good doctor. It takes a good head—and a good heart.

Appendix: Outline of the "Seminar in the Human Side of Medicine" Course at Macalester College

This is the outline of the course I taught at Macalester College in St. Paul, Minnesota. The limited enrollment of no more than fifteen students encourages reflective discussion and allows the students and me to get to know each other well.

SEMINAR IN THE HUMAN SIDE OF MEDICINE: WHAT IT'S LIKE TO BE A PATIENT; WHAT IT'S LIKE TO BE A PHYSICIAN

Laurence A. Savett, M D
Macalester College Department of Biology
Wednesday evenings, 7–9 p.m., 2 credit hours.

This course will concentrate on learning about how patients, their families, and professionals who care for them experience illness; how stories patients tell become the basis for diagnosis and therapeutic action; what it's like to be a physician; and the therapeutic relationship. Didactic presentations, interactive discussion using stories from patients', students', and the instructor's experiences, and related literature will provide the content of the course. Others, including faculty members, professional colleagues, and patients, will help provide material for our course work and participate in our discussions.

The Context of the Course

Two premises provide the basis for this course:

- If someone is to be a physician or other health care professional, it is as important to master the human dimensions as it is to master the mechanistic, biologic, and technical dimensions.
- The human side of medicine can be taught.

At a time when medicine is in transition and aspects of such a career that are most attractive to many prospective physicians relate to the technology of medicine, the community faces the hazard that the human side of medicine may be neglected. The human side of medicine includes a number of elements, among which are:

- A view of medicine encompassing biological, psychological, and social dimensions.
- Thoughtful medical history-taking techniques and ways to explore the psychological and social issues related to the patient's illness.
- The role of collaboration in medicine.
- The role of uncertainty in clinical medicine.
- The nature of the doctor-patient relationship.

What patients and their families ask for, and are entitled to, involves all of the above and includes competence in the technology of medicine in the context of a human approach to medical care. One or all of those factors may attract someone to a career in medicine, but the human side is often taught informally at best or "socialized out of" the student. When that happens, both the physician and the community lose. The physician misses out on those aspects that comprise some of the real joys of medicine, and the community of patients loses when its physicians lack the awareness of the importance of those dimensions.

Unless one is, by nature, a compassionate and understanding person, it is argued, the human side of medicine is difficult to teach. I believe it can be taught, and I believe that exposing undergraduates to those dimensions of a career in medicine should help to attract talented and compassionate people to such a career and provide a context and a head start for later learning in professional school. The community of patients is the ultimate beneficiary.

The Content of the Course

In this course, we will

1. Explore the experience of illness, starting with a detailed story of one patient's experience and stories of students' experiences and those of their families and friends, and asking other patients to describe to the students their own experiences with illness.
2. Explore what patients and their families expect from a physician.
3. Introduce the concept of "uncertainty" in medicine, how physicians, patients, and families deal with it, and how one can take action, despite the existence of uncertainty.
4. Look at the various ways patients and their families deal with illness.
5. Learn some of the methods of the medical interview as the primary means of gathering information about patients and the context in which their illnesses occur.
6. Introduce the concept of "differential diagnosis," the process by which physicians reason and make a diagnosis.
7. Explore the nuances of the doctor-patient relationship in order to illustrate that, beyond being a scientist and technician, the physician provides context, perspective, and emotional support for patients and their families.
8. Explore how a physician learns and ultimately becomes his or her own teacher.
9. Explore what the life of a physician is like and what physicians are like.

Methods

1. Each session will have many or all of the following dimensions:
   - A didactic portion.
   - Substantial discussion, using many stories and examples from students,' patients,' and the instructor's experiences.
   - A list of resources.
   - A look at how the lessons learned may have broader application.
   - Homework, exercises, and/or written assignments done in preparation for the session.
2. On most of your assignments, I will encourage you to work in pairs, to emphasize the concept that medicine is a collaborative profession and to illustrate many of the benefits of thoughtful collaboration.
3. Text and other material: We will use the extensive literature relating to the human side of medicine, patients' experiences, and uncertainty (see Selected Bibliography).

4. At the first session, we will discuss

   - Who the participants are.

   - Goals of the course, including what participants want from the course.

   - Collaboration.

   - Confidentiality.

   - The instructor's expectations of the participants.

5. There will no final exam. There will be a final paper on this subject: "Fashioning the best system of medical care possible: what would be ideal for the patient, what would be ideal for the physician." The content of the seminar should provide ample material for a thoughtful paper.

6. Your grade will be determined by the quality of your participation in seminar discussions and the quality of your written assignments and final paper. I believe the clarity with which you express yourself is a reflection of how you think. Part of the intent of the seminar is to enhance your ability to think and express yourself and to enhance your self-confidence in that ability.

7. Together we will have an opportunity to evaluate the seminar at the midpoint of the semester. At the end of the semester, you will have an opportunity to evaluate the course more completely.

I am looking forward to learning a great deal from each of you.

Course Outline

What It's Like to Be a Patient

Session I. Coronary artery bypass surgery: what one can learn from a patient and the patient's family. Introduction to the medical setting. The discussion will include

- Presentation of a way to look at each medical encounter as an opportunity to learn and to add to one's experience, in a five-step process that includes these questions:

  1. What is the *story?*
  2. What is the medical *history?*
  3. What are the *issues?*
  4. What is the role of the doctor-patient *relationship?*
  5. What did I *learn?*
- Introduction to the biopsychosocial model of medicine.

Session II. Seminar participants' experience with illness. The patient is the center of the drama.

Session III. How do people handle illness? Patients who have had serious illness will tell their stories and talk about how they dealt with their illness. Together we will address a number of themes: collaboration, the family experience of illness, and the role of physicians.

Session IV. Uncertainty. How patients, families, and physicians cope with uncertainty. The value of reason as a tool in diagnosis and treatment.

What It's Like to Be a Physician

Session V. The medical history. How stories patients tell become the basis for diagnosis and therapeutic action. What physicians need to know about illness. How to get patients to tell about themselves. What gets in the way of patients telling their stories.

Session VI. Diagnosis.

- *The differential diagnosis.* Giving a problem a name and then exploring the possible diagnostic solutions to the problem and the process by which a physician establishes a diagnosis.
- *The "problem-oriented system" of medical reasoning and decision making.* How to learn. How to become one's own teacher.

Session VII. What can go wrong.

- *Drug- and treatment-induced illness.* "First do no harm."
- *Prejudice.* Viewing people as members of a group rather than as individuals. What we can learn from examining prejudices. How to apply those lessons to patient care.
- *Abuse.*
- *Mistakes.*

Session VIII. Defining the issues. Unless all the issues are identified, the care of any patient may be inadequate and incomplete. The clearer the definition of the issues, the easier it is to address the problems, and "a problem identified is a problem half solved."

Session IX. Medicine is a collaborative profession. During this session, a physician, a social worker, a nurse, and a hospital chaplain will collaborate with the patient and the patient's family, help clarify and enlarge the story and the clinical history, identify the issues, and show how the relationship with the patient and the patient's family can facilitate care.

Session X. What is a professional? Four people, none of them in health care, all "real professionals," will describe their work and talk about what they do that makes them professionals. With them we will explore the professional dimensions common to their diverse careers and apply what we have learned to the "professional" quality of a medical career.

Session XI. The different faces of physicians. Three physicians will describe their professional lives and how they integrate their professional and personal lives. The role of values. Dealing with change.

The Doctor-Patient Relationship

Session XII. The doctor-patient relationship. What patients expect from physicians. How the doctor-patient relationship is like the teacher-student relationship. The importance of the relationship to the patient *and* to the physician.

Summing Up

Session XIII. What have we learned about physicians, patients, families, teaching and learning, and choosing a career. The transition from "learning about a patient" to "learning from a patient." Fashioning the best system possible: what would be ideal for the patient, what would be ideal for the physician.

Notes

INTRODUCTION

1. *Pirke Avot*, Chapter 2, Mishnah 16. *Pirke Avot* is an early second-century collection of rabbinic law and thought.

2. Adin Steinsalz, *The Talmud, the Steinsalz Edition* (New York: Random House, 1989), p. 4.

3. Ibid., p. 9.

CHAPTER 1

1. Quoted also as "80 percent of success is 'showing up'" in *Current Biographies 1966*, and *American Behavioral Scientist*, 1977 (Mar./Apr.), Vol. 10, No. 5: 672,

CHAPTER 2

1. Thomas Lynch, *The Undertaking* (New York: W. W. Norton and Company, 1997), p. 97.

CHAPTER 3

1. L.A. Savett, Spirituality and Practice: Stories, Barriers and Opportunities. *Creative Nursing.* 1997; No. 4: 7–11, 16.

CHAPTER 4

1. Anatole Broyard, *Intoxicated by My Illness* (New York: Fawcett Columbine, 1992), p. 44.

2. Ibid., p. 42.

3. Robertson Davies, *The Cunning Man* (New York: Viking Penguin, 1995), p. 245.

4. Broyard, *Intoxicated by My Illness*, p. 55.

CHAPTER 6

1. For the validation of my reflections many years ago and for the additional stimulation to think more completely about these issues, I am indebted to conversations with Harold Bursztajn, M.D., and to the book he co-authored: H. Bursztajn, R. Feinbloom, R. Hamm, and A. Brodsky. *Medical Choices, Medical Chances: How Patients, Families and Physicians Can Cope with Uncertainty* (New York: Delacorte Press, 1981). Some of the material in this chapter has been presented in another form in L.A. Savett. Dealing with Uncertainty: Yet Another Dimension of Caring for Our Patients. *Creative Nursing.* 1995 (Jan./Feb.); Vol. 1, Issue 3: 11–13, 20.

2. Mike Augustin, "Twins Blast Bosox, 8-2" in *St. Paul Sunday Pioneer Press*, 1979 (June 3); Sec. F: p. 1.

3. Jacob Bronowski, *The Ascent of Man* (Boston: Little, Brown and Company, 1973), p. 360.

CHAPTER 8

1. Richard Scarry, *Richard Scarry's What Do People Do All Day?* (New York: Random House, 1968).

CHAPTER 9

1. The full quote, from Emile Gruppé, a premier Cape Ann, Massachusetts, artist, is "Painting is like story-telling. No two people tell a story the same way. That's what makes art so interesting." The quote was displayed during the exhibit, "Emile Gruppé and His Contemporaries," August 2–31, 1997, at the North Shore Art Association, Gloucester, Massachusetts.

2. Marian R. Stuart and Joseph A. Lieberman, *The Fifteen Minute Hour* (New York: Praeger Publishers, 1986), pp. 102–103. The title of the book, a play on the traditional "fifty-minute hour" of the psychiatrist's session with a patient, indicates that a physician can use well-chosen questions to learn a great deal about a patient in a short period of time.

3. Robertson Davies, *The Cunning Man* (New York: Viking Penguin, 1995), p. 97.

CHAPTER 10

1. First described by Lawrence Weed, M.D., my teacher at Cleveland Metropolitan General Hospital, the problem-oriented system has had a profound impact on how a whole generation of physicians has practiced and taught. See L.L. Weed, Medical Records That Guide and Teach. *New England Journal of Medicine*. 1978; Vol. 256: 593–600 (Part 1), 652–657 (Part 2).

CHAPTER 12

1. From L.A. Savett, Values: Personal and Professional. *Creative Nursing*. 2000; Vol. 6, Issue 3: 3.

2. Douglas Wood, D.O., Ph.D., used this definition in a talk on June 28, 2000, at the biennial convention of the National Association of Advisors to the Health Professions in Orlando, Florida.

3. Robertson Davies, *The Cunning Man* (New York: Viking Penguin, 1994), p. 245.

4. Secretary of State Dean Acheson described his working relationship with President Harry Truman in this way in David McCullough, *Truman* (New York: Simon and Schuster, 1992), p. 752.

5. Most of the material in this section was originally published in L.A. Savett and S.G. Savett. Genuine Collaboration: Our Obligation to Our Patients and To Each Other. *Creative Nursing*. 1994 (Sept./Oct.), 11–13.

6. My wife, who co-authored the original article containing this story, and I are grateful to our friend, teacher, and model, Annie Laurie Baker, for allowing us to tell part of her story. For many years, Ms. Baker was director of the Department of Social Service at the University of Minnesota Hospitals.

CHAPTER 13

1. H. Bursztajn, R. Feinbloom, R. Hamm and A. Brodsky, *Medical Choices, Medical Chances: How Patients, Families, and Physicians Can Cope with Uncertainty* (New York: Delacorte Press, 1981), pp. xv–xvi.

CHAPTER 14

1. Arthur Frank, *At the Will of the Body* (Boston: Houghton Mifflin, 1991), p. 14.

2. Philip Roth, *Patrimony* (New York: Simon and Schuster, 1991), p. 233.

3. Adapted from H. Bursztajn, R.I. Feinbloom, R.H. Hamm, and A. Brodsky, *Medical Choices, Medical Chances: How Patients, Families, and Physicians Can Cope with Uncertainty*. (New York: Delacorte Press, 1981), pp. 3–19.

4. The exhibit, "Minnesota Communities," ran from October 1993 until October 1998 at the Minnesota Historical Society, St. Paul, Minnesota.

CHAPTER 15

1. This section is adapted from L.A. Savett, Drug-Induced Illness: Causes for Delayed Diagnosis and a Strategy for Early Recognition. *Postgraduate Medicine.* 1980; Vol. 67: 155–166. The two cases described are, respectively, Cases 4 and 14 from that article.

2. From *The American Heritage Dictionary of the English Language* (New York: American Heritage Publishing Co., 1971), p. 1,033.

3. Much of this section is adapted from L.A. Savett, Medical Care and Teaching: Stories of Inadequacy, Opportunities for Growth. *Primarily Nursing.* 1994 (Jan./Feb.); Vol. 8, Issue 1: 10–12.

4. *American Heritage Dictionary,* p. 6.

5. Henry Louis Gates, "Powell and the Black Elite." *New Yorker.* 1995 (Sept. 25); 64–65.

6. David Hilfiker, "Mistakes," in eds., R. Reynold and J. Stone, *On Doctoring.* (New York: Simon and Schuster, 1995), pp. 379, 392.

7. Ibid., pp. 375–376.

CHAPTER 16

1. James Agate, a British drama critic and novelist (1877–1947), wrote this in his diary, July 19, 1945. Quoted in *The Oxford Dictionary of Quotations,* 5th edition, E. Knowles, ed. (Oxford, U.K.: Oxford University Press, 1999), p. 6.

2. From *How to Abandon Ship,* a 1942 handbook for merchant seamen, cited in editorial "Setting the Sextant Aside." *New York Times.* 1998 (May 22); Sec. A: 24.

CHAPTER 17

1. An earlier version of this chapter was originally published as L.A. Savett, Values and Dealing with Change. *Creative Nursing.* 2000; Vol. 6, Issue 3: 11–14.

2. See frontispiece.

3. Interview with Paul Newman on the television program, "Inside the Actors' Studio," broadcast on Bravo Channel, July 21, 1996.

4. Arthur Kleinman, *The Illness Narratives. Suffering, Healing, and the Human Condition* (New York: Basic Books, 1988), pp. 209–226.

CHAPTER 18

1. Chaim Potok, *In the Beginning* (New York: Alfred A. Knopf, 1975), p. 3.

2. Thanks to Gregory Plotnikoff, M.D., for this insight.

3. Batya Gur, *The Saturday Morning Murder* (New York: HarperCollins Publishers, 1993), p. 61.

CHAPTER 19

1. William Shakespeare. *As You Like It*, Act II, scene vii, verse 138.

2. *Enhanced autonomy*, a term introduced by Timothy Quill in T.E. Quill, "Physician recommendations and patient autonomy: Finding a balance between physician power and patient choice." *Annals of Internal Medicine* 125: 763–769, 1996.

3. Jon Pratt, *Foundation Grants 1999 Factbook*. p. 57. Based in Minneapolis, Pratt is the director of a consortium of non-profit organizations.

CHAPTER 20

1. Robertson Davies, *The Cunning Man* (New York: Viking Penguin, 1995), pp. 246–247.

2. Mary Twelveponies, *There Are No Problem Horses, Only Problem Riders* (Boston: Houghton Mifflin Co., 1982).

3. Robert Coles, *The Call of Stories* (Boston: Houghton Mifflin Co., 1989), p. 8.

CHAPTER 21

1. Anatole Broyard, *Intoxicated by My Illness* (New York: Fawcett Columbine, 1992), pp. 40, 45.

2. Much of this section appeared in L.A. Savett, How Can I Keep from Becoming Emotionally Involved? *Creative Nursing*. 1998; Vol. 4: 3–5. It was also presented in a talk to first-year medical students at the University of Minnesota on October 1, 1998.

3. Robert Coles, *The Call of Stories* (Boston: Houghton Mifflin Co., 1989), p. 9.

4. Broyard, *Intoxicated by My Illness*, p. 49.

5. Anne Lamott, *Bird by Bird* (New York: Pantheon, 1994), p. 179.

CHAPTER 23

1. Chaim Potok, *In the Beginning* (New York: Alfred A. Knopf, 1975), p. 3.

2. Previously reported in L.A. Savett, Medical Care and Teaching: Stories of Inadequacy, Opportunities for Growth. *Primarily Nursing*. 1994 (Jan./Feb.); Vol. 8, Issue 1: 10–12.

3. Blanche Wiesen Cook, *Eleanor Roosevelt, Vol. 1, 1884–1933* (New York: Viking Penguin, 1992), p. 8.

4. Pirke Avot, Chapter 4, Mishnah 1. *Pirke Avot* is an early second-century collection of rabbinic law and thought.

5. Whitey Herzog, *You're Missing a Great Game* (New York: Simon and Schuster, 1999), p. 2.

6. Theodore Bikel, *Theo: The Autobiography of Theodore Bikel* (New York: Harper Collins, 1994), p. 319.

7. From the obituary of my former teacher, Paul Yu, M.D., *Times Union*, Rochester, N.Y., 1991, May 22; sec. B: p. 8. Also quoted as "If you plan for a year, plant a seed. If for ten years, plant a tree. If for a hundred years, teach the people." In Kuan Chung, *Kuan-Tzu (Book of Master Kuan)—Kuan Tzu Chi P'ing.* Ed. Ling Ju-heng, 1970, vol. 1, p. 12.

Selected Bibliography

Each of these books has been a resource for my course. I encourage students to read specific sections or chapters in preparation for their papers and class discussions and then to read the rest at their leisure. I also encourage the students to talk over the content with a learning partner. The readers of this book can do the same.

All of these are in paperback. *Intoxicated by My Illness* (Broyard) and *Medical Choices, Medical Chances* (Bursztajn et al.) are now out of print.

Broyard, Anatole. *Intoxicated by My Illness*. New York: Fawcett Columbine, 1992. The former editor of the *New York Times* Book Review section provides an account of his own illness and reflects on the physician-patient relationship.

Bursztajn, Harold; Feinbloom, Richard; Hamm, Robert; and Brodsky, Archie. *Medical Choices, Medical Chances: How Patients, Families, and Physicians Can Cope with Uncertainty*. New York: Delacorte Press, 1981. The authors describe the importance of acknowledging uncertainty in medicine and strategies for dealing with it.

Coles, Robert. *The Call of Stories*. Boston: Houghton Mifflin Co., 1989. Dr. Coles, a psychiatrist, teaches Harvard undergraduates and medical and other graduate students about the lessons we can learn from listening to patients'—and each other's—stories.

Colgrove, Melba; Bloomfield, Harold; and McWilliams, Peter. *How to Survive the Loss of a Love*. Los Angeles: Prelude Press, 1976. A physician, a psychologist, and a poet present insights about loss for patients and for professionals and others involved in their care.

Fadiman, Anne. *The Spirit Catches You and You Fall Down*. New York: Noonday Press, 1997. In presenting the story of the illness of a Hmong patient who has been inserted into the American medical culture, the author describes the consequences of the cultural clash for her and her family's care.

Kleinman, Arthur. *The Illness Narratives: Suffering, Healing, and the Human Condition*. New York: Basic Books, Inc., 1988. A physician presents stories of illness and their meaning to patients and families and describes different ways in which physicians deal with patients and with change.

Remen, Rachel Naomi. *Kitchen Table Wisdom*. New York, Riverhead Books, 1996; and *My Grandfather's Blessings. Stories of Strength, Refuge, and Belonging*. New York: Riverhead Books, 2000. Using stories from her own practice, a physician who specializes in caring for patients with serious or chronic illness reflects on how she has used what she has learned from her experience in each new therapeutic relationship.

Verghese, Abraham. *My Own Country*. New York: Simon and Schuster, 1994. A physician specializing in infectious diseases writes of his experience in caring for patients with AIDS in rural Tennessee and its impact on his personal life.

Index

About the Author

LAURENCE A. SAVETT, M.D. practiced primary care internal medicine in Gloucester, Massachusetts, and St. Paul, Minnesota, for 30 years. Dr. Savett teaches about the psychological and social dimensions of medicine and the doctor-patient relationship at the University of Minnesota Medical School, where he is Clinical Professor of Medicine, and at Macalester College and the University of St. Thomas, where he helps advise pre-medical and other pre-health professional students. He has served on the admissions committee of the University of Minnesota Medical School and the board on the Central Region of the National Association of Advisors for the Health Professions. He is a Fellow of the American College of Physicians.

CPSIA information can be obtained
at www.ICGtesting.com
Printed in the USA
FSOW01n2344210117
29892FS

9 780865 693197